The
Psychedelic
Garden

DISCLAIMER

Royal Botanic Gardens **Kew**

The
Psychedelic
Garden

Mind-altering plants in folklore, superstition and popular culture

Sandra Lawrence

WELBECK

Introduction

In 1957, while writing to his friend Aldous Huxley, the radical English psychiatrist Humphry Fortescue Osmond found himself stumped for a term to describe substances that produce hallucinogenic effects in the human brain. He eventually combined two Greek words: *psyche* (mind) and *delos* (manifest).

Osmond's term, *psychedelic*, has been with us ever since, though the man himself was highly suspicious of the 1960s counterculture his word would later epitomize. He regarded such compounds as mysterious, maybe even dangerous, but was fascinated by their potential. Others have been equally inspired, including social reformers, political activists and, perhaps above all, artists.

In many cultures plants with psychoactive properties are considered sacred. They are sentient beings, divine teachers, certainly not "drugs". It can be disconcerting to juxtapose the sincerity of an indigenous ceremony involving the likes of peyote, psilocybin or ayahuasca with the casual, recreational use the same substances often acquire in the Global North.

For some, the psychedelic world can be scary. Who knows what images our brains might conjure if we were to lose control? It becomes even more unnerving when we realize that Science (with a capital "S") does not fully understand these plants either. We can isolate individual chemicals, but even within a single species there may be several compounds which may react according to outside influences, including geographical or meteorological conditions. A plant that has lived in the sunshine at the top of a mountain can develop different amounts of certain compounds to the same species living in dark, wet rainforest at the mountain's base. Further complications arise when two or more plants are combined, and the effects of such brews vary yet again according to each individual. Indigenous peoples have known this for centuries, but for Western medicine, used to prescribing one drug for one ailment, it is nothing short of alchemy.

Not all mind-altering plants are psychedelic, of course. This book also explores everyday stimulants – tea, coffee and nicotine, for example – alongside depressants such as alcohol and cannabis, and addictive "hard drugs", including opium and cocaine.

Plants are not the only source of psychotropic compounds. I have had to leave out psychedelic fish, toads, sea sponges, "mad honey" and lab-born synthetics. I have also omitted psychoactive photosynthetic eukaryotes, for the prosaic but practical reason that, inexplicably, there is little folklore about algae. I have, however, included fungi, using the feeble excuse that, until very recently, mushrooms were considered part of the plant kingdom.

Then there is the art, the music, the literature and popular culture, which, even more than other titles in this series, is crucial to the way we approach these plants. The stories we tell ourselves about drugs, whatever the medium, end up as tangled as the webs famously spun by spiders given various psychedelics by Swiss pharmacologist Peter Witt, but they may just be the best roadmap we have to understanding the complex world of substance-induced altered states.

Sandra Lawrence

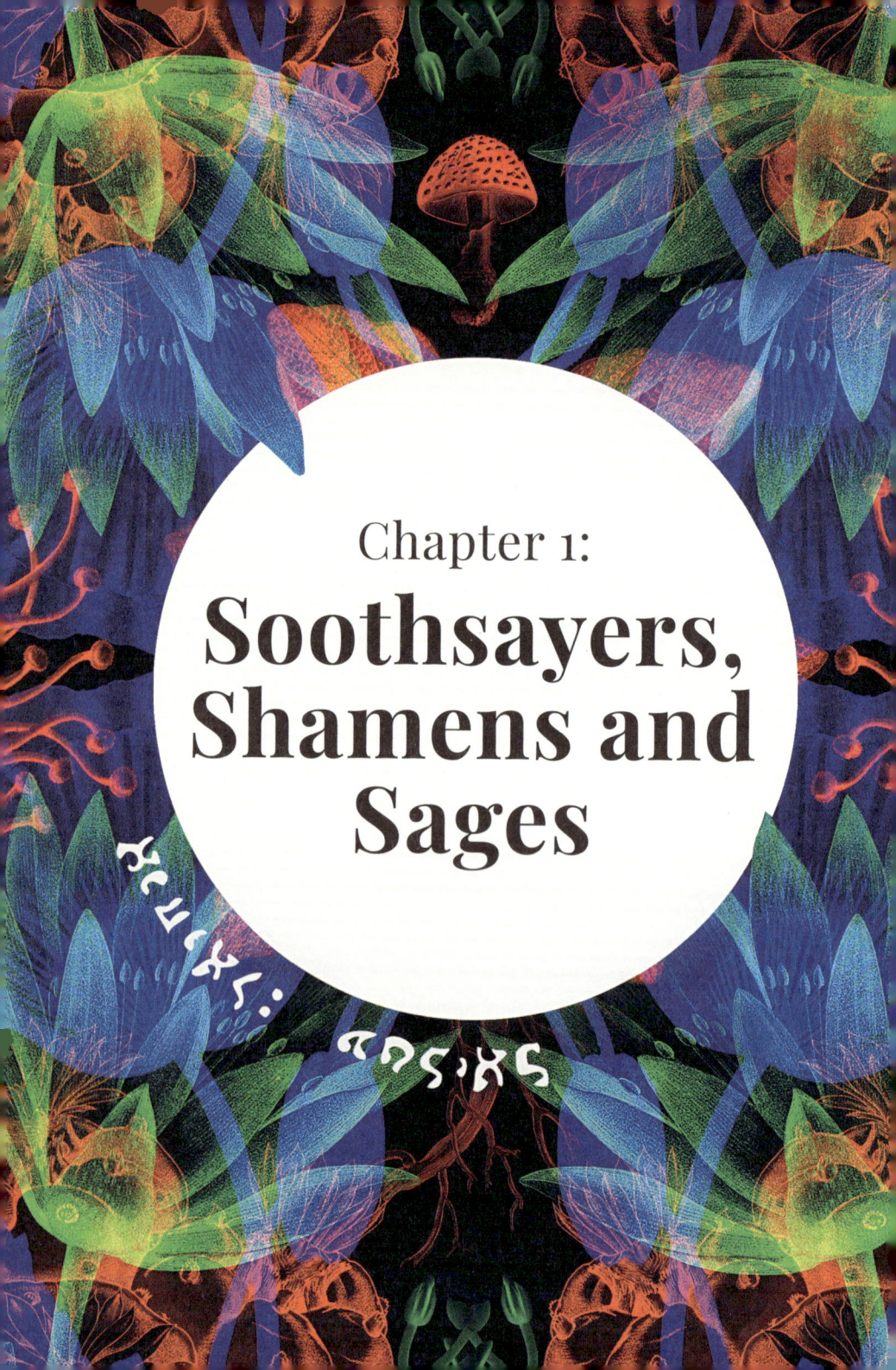

Chapter 1:
Soothsayers, Shamens and Sages

The vast natural caves at Es Càrritx in Menorca contain the last resting places of more than 200 Bronze Age individuals dating from between 1400 BCE and 800 BCE. Analysis of hair strands found in tiny receptacles reveal the presence of psychotropic substances atropine, scopolamine and ephedrine found in local plants such as mandrake (*Mandragora autumnalis*), devil's snare (*Datura stramonium*), henbane (*Hyoscyamus albus*) and joint pine (*Ephedra fragilis*). Were these people the world's first psychonauts? Probably not…

Kaleidoscopic Lights in our Darkest Pasts

Archaeologists believe humans were using San Pedro cactus in Peru as far back as 8600 BCE. Traces of cannabis clinging to pottery discovered at Okinoshima, Japan date to around 8200 BCE. They, too, however, are by no means alone.

Whether coca in Peru, betel in Thailand, waterlilies in Egypt or psilocybin mushrooms in Guatemala, humans appear to have been entirely aware of – and actively using – mind-altering substances since our species began. Barely a month goes by without another excavation revealing new evidence: perhaps pollen samples, pictographs or a ceramic figurine clutching a sacred mushroom; perhaps microscopic remains of the plants themselves or even paraphernalia not dissimilar to that used today.

What we are less clear about is how such plants were used. We are quick to assume our ancestors had ritual, spiritual or medicinal purposes for them, but if a substance was enjoyable, might people have enjoyed it recreationally too?

We have no idea, for example, what went on at the annual Eleusinian Mysteries, celebratory festivals dedicated to the goddess Demeter between 1600 BCE and 392 CE. This is because, on pain of death, the first rule of the Eleusinian Mysteries was that no one talked about the Eleusinian Mysteries. Participants allegedly drank *kykeon*, usually a mixture of water, barley, goat cheese and herbs, but scholars

hypothesize that at the Mysteries the beverage acquired another ingredient: the psychoactive fungus ergot. It's not impossible. Recent excavations have revealed ergot remains in a ceremonial drinking vessel dedicated to Demeter, and in the dental calculus of a 25-year-old man from 300 BCE. Was the celebration spiritual, mystical, recreational or all three? We will likely never know.

We can be a little surer about substances that have a modern-day equivalent. A thousand-year-old leather bag found in the Cueva del Chileno rock shelter in the Bolivian Andes once held wood and bone equipment to crush the seeds of psychoactive plants, along with a snuffing tube, and a pouch made from the snouts of three Andean foxes. This contained traces of at least five psychoactive substances, all ingredients for the hallucinogenic drink ayahuasca, still very much revered today.

While the ritual and spiritual use of psychoactive plants has apparently enjoyed a relatively unbroken line among certain indigenous cultures, historical paths in Western history are less clear. Some intoxicants were constants. Alcohol, created when organic substances are fermented into beer and wine, or distilled as spirits, has always been with us. Caffeine arrived in early modern Europe in the form of coffee, tea and cocoa. Tobacco was brought from the New World, then distributed to the rest

Opposite A drawing of Xochiquetzal, the Aztec goddess of beauty, fertility, love and flowers.

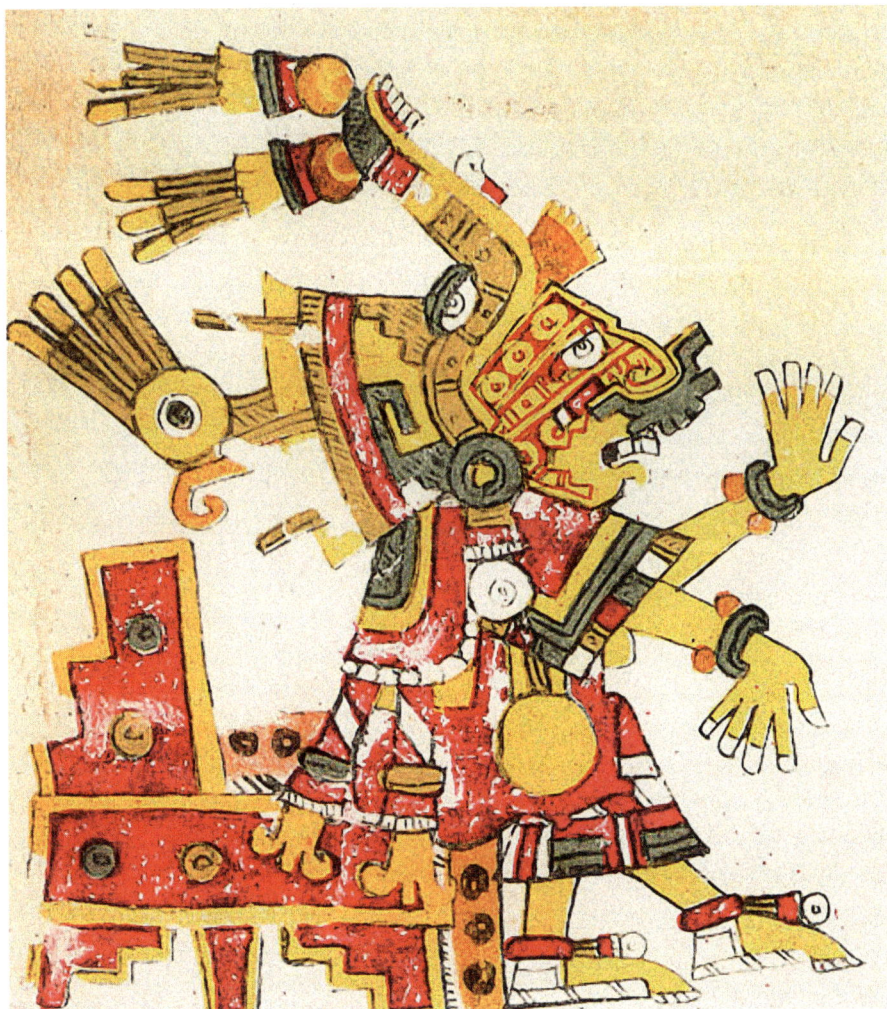

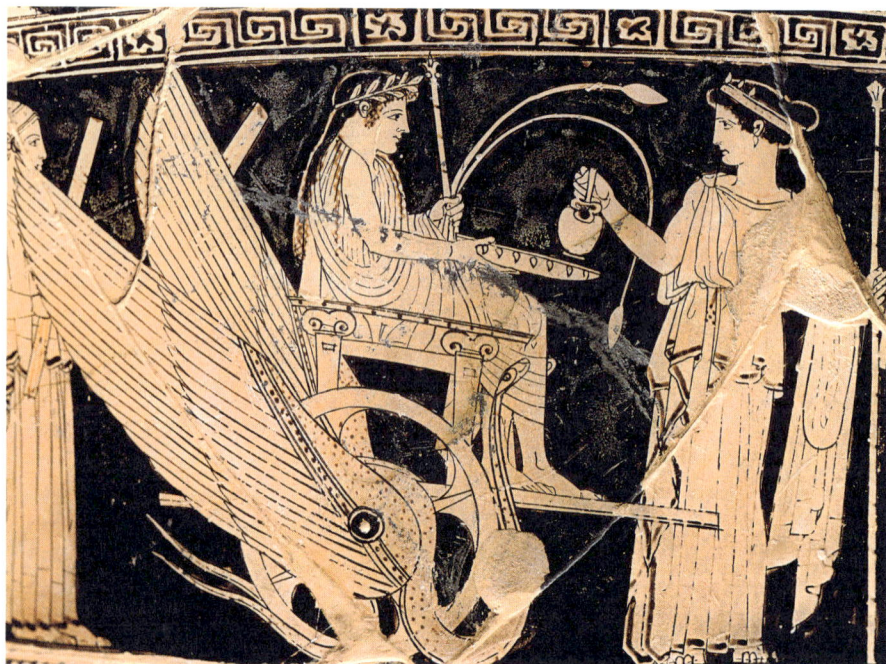

Above A scene from a piece of pottery dated 460BC, showing Triptolemus, who is worshipped as the patron of agriculture, in a winged chariot next to Demeter.

of the planet. Sugar, not always considered mind-altering, but which some have claimed to be the most addictive substance of all, moved from being a rare treat to a commodity as vast sugar cane plantations were established from the sixteenth century onwards.

But what of the classic drugs that will take up most of the pages in this book? The opiates, the narcotics, the hallucinogens? Some were cultivated for medicinal uses; for example, opium was grown in Mesopotamia in the third millennium BCE, spreading to ancient Egypt and Greece, arriving in the rest of Europe between the tenth and thirteenth century.

Others were noted poisons, their mind-altering properties whispered about as the work of the Devil (see the Hexing Herbs, p. 162), used only by physicians and carefully warned against in herbals and religious treatises alike. In South and Central America, Jesuit missionaries wrote extensively of horrors they witnessed watching "natives" ingesting strange substances that conjured satanic visions and crazed behaviour.

Things began to change in the early nineteenth century as chemists worked to isolate compounds within plants and experiment with their possible uses. After millennia of pain, the human race finally found true relief as wonder drugs such as morphine and cocaine hit the market, albeit entirely uncontrolled, leading to a heady but extremely dangerous zenith. The only way was down. Even as people began to understand the dangers, they realized that some of these miracles were highly addictive.

Western botanists had begun travelling in earnest to areas of the world previously unexplored (by Europeans), searching for "undiscovered" plants, both ornamental and useful. Richard Spruce was one of several "plant hunters" sent to the Amazon rainforest by the Royal Botanic Gardens, Kew in the 1850s. Collecting as many samples as he could, Spruce did not partake of the indigenous ayahuasca ceremonies he also witnessed among the people he encountered there, but he would inspire others such as Richard Evans Schultes (see p. 138), who realized that the only way to understand such plants was to learn from the people already familiar with them.

Things were moving fast. In the early twentieth century, the Western world was in new pain, both physical and psychological, from a combination of war, pandemic and economic depression. The narcotics cat was well and truly out of the bag – used,

as ever, for medicinal and emotional purposes but also, increasingly, for reasons creative, recreational or philosophical or, more darkly, because the user could not stop.

As psychoactive, and especially entheogenic substances became ever more varied, even synthesized, the stories we told ourselves about them changed, too. Drugs were "evil", screamed the headlines but, like all bad things, they were alluring, too. They were everywhere: in novels, films, music, art, and even our own personal rituals, and they've stayed there. Whether indulging in that innocent pick-me-up cup of tea, first cigarette of the day, occasional psychedelic mushroom trip or pipe full of freshly cooked crack, for better or worse, mind-altering substances are now part of our world.

Below A Mayan carving of a chieftan, eagle and snake from Chichen Itza, Yucatan, Mexico.

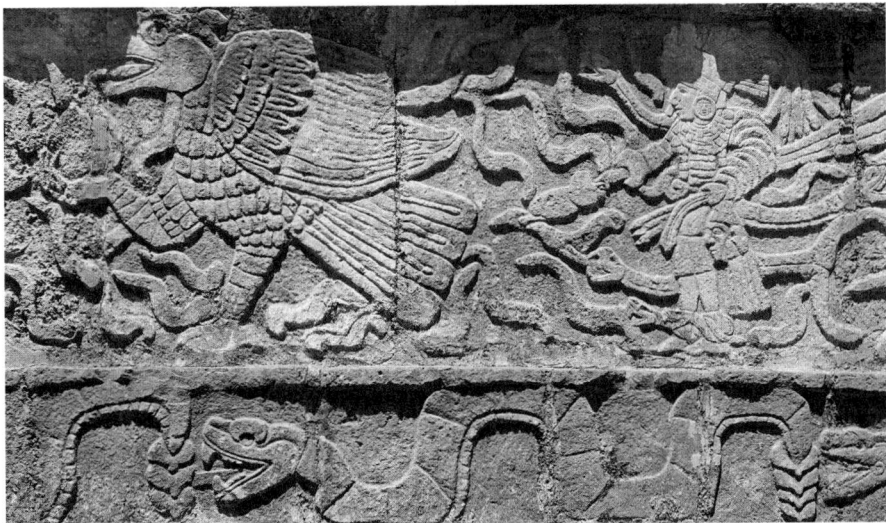

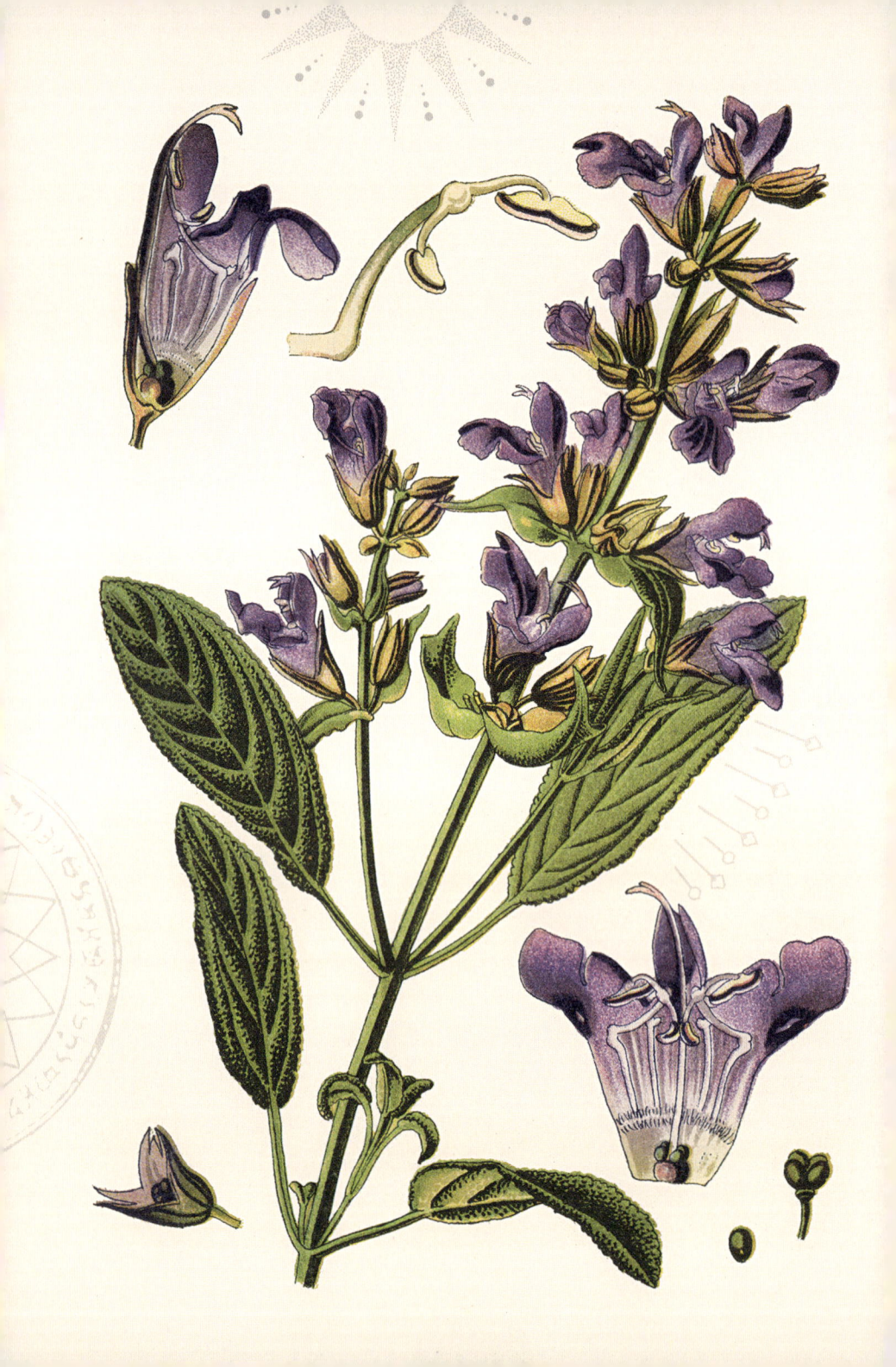

Diviner's sage

Salvia divinorum

In 2007 a spate of videos featuring teenagers smoking "something", then laughing like maniacs and crashing into things, unable to coordinate the simplest movements, caused a worldwide panic, particularly in the United States.

Horrified news anchors, senators and legislators were quick to denounce the "diviner's sage" and when a suicide of an American teenager was linked to the drug, new countries joined the list of nations already controlling the substance. The videos shocked the plant's original users too, but for different reasons. The Mazatec people of Oaxaca, Mexico have a profound respect for the plant and were mortified to see it being used for trivial purposes.

Despite its name, diviner's or seer's sage has nothing to do with oracles or soothsayers of ancient Greece. *S. divinorum* is a member of the mint family (and is sometimes called magic mint), and unlike the sun-loving common sage (*S. officinalis*), it loves the shady, subtropical cloud forests of Central America. It contains salvinorin A, a potent psychotropic molecule.

The plant, also known as *yerba de la pastora* (shepherd's herb), had been used for centuries but was unknown to science until 1939, when anthropologist Jean Bassett Johnson visited the Mazatec to study shamanism. The Global North had to wait until 1962 to see a live plant, collected by R. Gordon Wasson and Albert Hofmann. Excited, Wasson suggested it could be the mythical Aztec plant *pipiltzintzintli* (Pure Prince). Hofmann was less happy with its scientific name, complaining that *Salvia divinorum* meant "sage of the ghosts" and that it should be *Salvia divinatorum*, "sage of the priests".

The Mazatec ceremony is serene, trance-like, slow, usually held at night. Male and female shamans work with questors – the sick, the victims of witchcraft or robbery, or those who just need guidance. They brew a tea, or twist fresh leaves (thirteen pairs is ideal) into a "quid" (lump) and chew slowly while the psychoactive substances are absorbed in the mouth. Chewing fresh leaves can produce quite strong visions but if swallowed, the stomach's gastric juices can "deactivate" the salvinorin A, to influence the plant's hallucinogenic properties.

Salvinorin A is classed as a dissociative hallucinogen, distorting perception and bringing an otherworldly, movie-like sense of detachment, especially when the leaves are dried for smoking.

Diviner's sage is not considered an addictive drug (for many, once is more than enough), but high doses can induce psychosis or depression, and for this reason it is banned in many countries, states, and in all U.S. Army bases.

Betel

Areca catechu;
Piper betle

A Vietnamese legend tells of twin brothers, the oldest of
whose wife mistook the younger brother for her husband and
welcomed him into her bed.

Immediately after the liaison, the brother was
consumed with shame. He left the village
and killed himself and was instantly turned
to limestone. The older brother went in search of
his twin. Finding the rock, he died of grief and was
transformed into a slender *Areca catechu* palm
tree. The wife followed the brothers and on finding
the stone and tree, became a creeping betel vine,
clinging to her husband's trunk for eternity.

The story explains the way *Piper betle* leaves are
used to wrap seeds from the areca palm (confusingly
called betel nuts) with lime and other ingredients,
including cardamom, cloves and, occasionally,
tobacco, to make a preparation called betel or
paan. The resulting quid has a bitter, peppery taste
and works as a mild stimulant, bringing a slightly
heightened awareness and generally warm sensation
to the chewer. The main alkaloid in betel nut (*Areca
catechu*) is arecoline, which has some similar
psychoactive and addictive effects to nicotine.

Chewing betel stimulates large quantities of
saliva, which turns red. The resulting stains around
the mouth, and especially the teeth, have enabled
archaeologists to date the practice to at least 2680
BCE and a group of pink-jawed skeletons in Duyong
Cave on Palawan Island in the Philippines. The habit

spread across Asia, where an estimated 400 million
people still indulge today. The mixture is unpleasant
to swallow and is usually spat out – whether this
is into a receptacle or onto the floor depends on
individual cultures. Even less pleasant side effects
may be seen in betel's growing links with oral
and oesophageal cancers (which increase when
combined with tobacco), heart disease, asthma,
stroke, stillbirth and premature babies with low
birth weights.

Despite these drawbacks, it is hard to understate
the social, spiritual and medical importance of betel.
In Ayurvedic medicine, which seeks to balance the
body, betel is considered a "cool" plant; areca is
"hot". Betel is believed by many to aid digestion, clear
phlegm, sweeten breath and remove tapeworms.
The Malaysian city Penang even takes its name from
pinang, Malay for "betel", and incorporates an areca
palm into its flag.

For Hindus, areca belongs to Brahma the
creator; the betel leaf is associated with Vishnu, the
preserver. Women offer each other a combination
of the two in colourful baskets during pujas (ritual
prayers) to invite Vishnu's consort Lakshmi into their
homes. Such gifts are very auspicious, and brides
are sometimes offered a single areca nut to add to

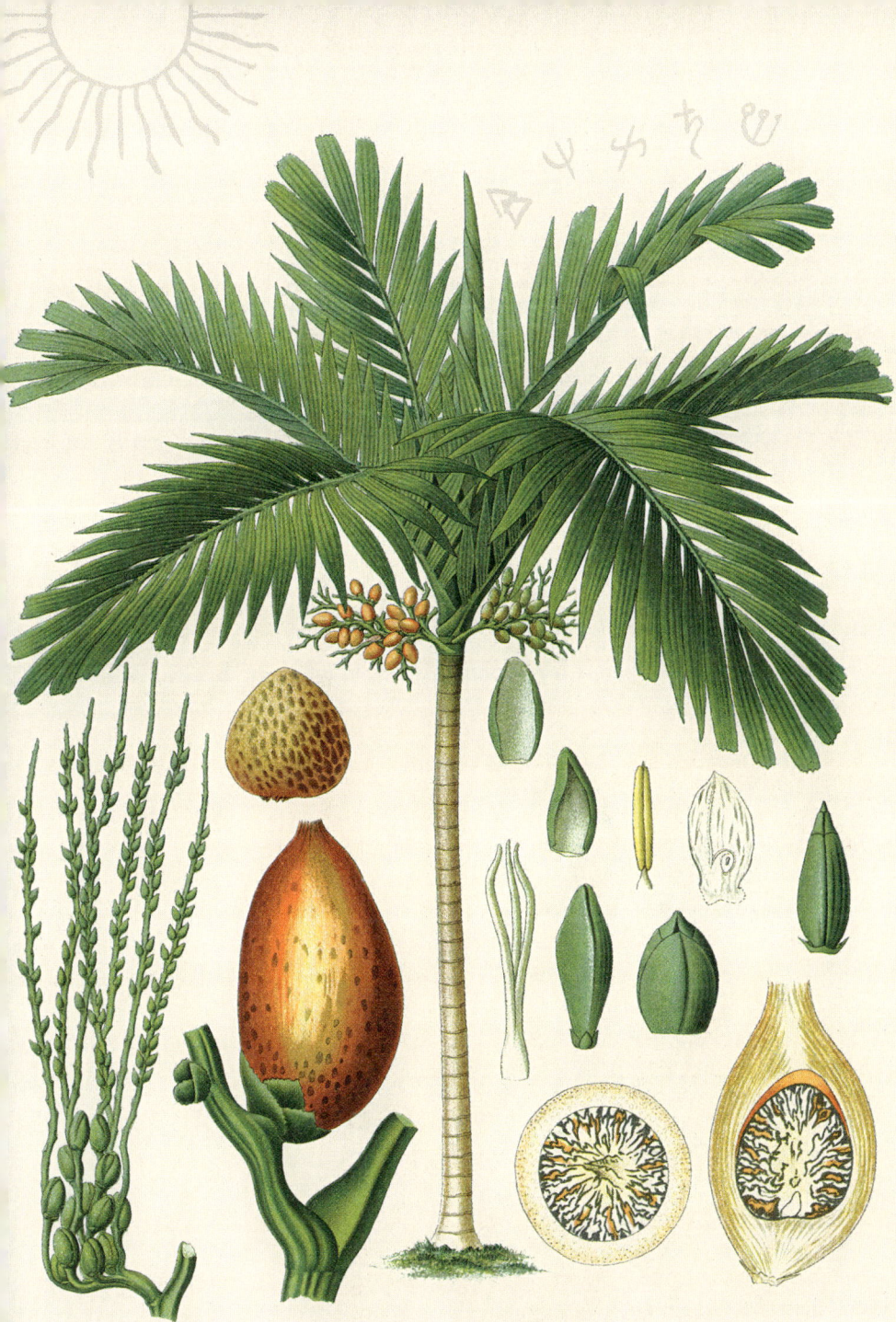

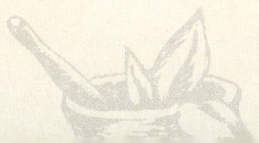

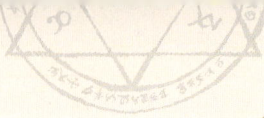

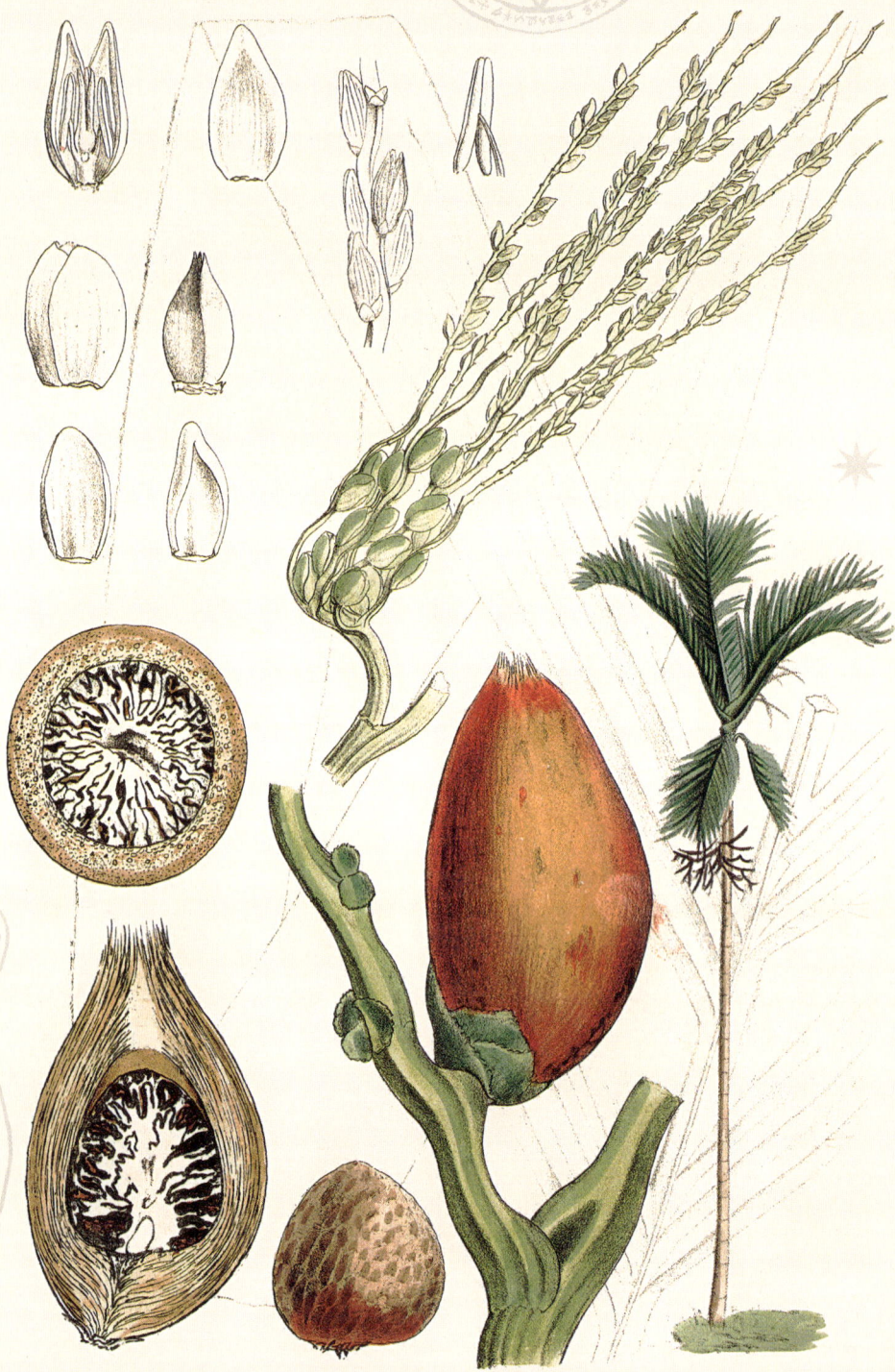

the ten heart-shaped betel leaves they carry to their wedding. Betel is also associated with the ape deity Hanuman who, in the *Ramayana*, visited Rama's abducted wife. Sita was delighted but had only betel to offer him. Devotees still hang garlands of the leaves around his statue.

Royalty stored betel in highly decorated boxes of gold, silver, tortoiseshell and ivory, expectorating into equally ornate spittoons, but more often, betel represents equality in hospitality.

In Meghalaya the Khasi people tell of two childhood friends, one rich, one poor. The rich man entertained his friend lavishly, and the poor man felt he should reciprocate. On the day of the visit, however, there was no food in the house. Feeling ashamed, the poor man and his wife took their own lives. Arriving, the rich man killed himself too, for failing to notice his friend's pain. A robber broke in and, finding three corpses, also died by suicide in case he was implicated in their deaths. In memory of all four, the custom of sharing *kwai* (betel) became egalitarian. The areca seed represents the rich man; the lime paste and leaf, the poor husband. The secret place between the lip and gum is where Khasi women hide the quid from the thief. Even poor households offer kwai to guests on arrival and after meals. When someone in Meghalaya dies, they are said to have gone to take kwai with God.

By contrast, if you are talking about "matters of betel and areca" in Vietnam, you are referring to marriage. The nut (male) and leaf (female) symbolize love, and the first "business" meeting between the parents of a prospective bride and groom begins with their chewing betel together.

Taiwanese construction workers, long-distance lorry drivers and fishermen often chew betel to stave off hunger pangs and stay awake across long hours, purchasing supplies from "Betel Nut Beauties". Many consider the practice of scantily clad young female vendors waiting in neon-lit, glass-walled roadside booths exploitative; others argue it empowers otherwise poor women to stay self-sufficient.

Betel has a much darker side: black magic. For some years baseball players of the Amis people in Taiwan accused their Puyuma rivals of casting evil spells on matches by burying cursed areca nuts to skew the results. Bead-strung seeds were found under the pitch, but their purpose is fiercely debated, and some suggest the controversy was based in negative tribal stereotyping, deliberately misunderstanding the magical importance conferred by Puyuma people on the areca. One thing is clear: betel is one of the most socially complex psychoactive plant combinations in the world.

Shamanism

Fewer than 70,000 people speak the Manchu–Tungus languages, stretched across vast regions between China and Russia, including Mongolia and Siberia, yet they have given the world one of its most evocative nouns.

The word *ša* means "to know", so a *šaman* is literally "one who knows". Probably introduced to Europe by the seventeenth-century Dutch traveller Nicolaas Witsen, the term has been stretched by anthropologists to embrace "ones who know" within many indigenous communities centred around animism: the belief that that the human world is surrounded by invisible spirits. These include Arctic, Native American, South and Central American, Australian Aboriginal and some African cultures. Shamans – extraordinary people of any gender, some still using an old, feminized form, *shamanka* – have one thing in common: they work via the medium of ecstatic trance, often using hallucinogenic substances gathered from the natural world.

Their roles vary, even between villages, but include functions roughly equating to healer, priest, counsellor, communicator and interceptor between regular people and the spirits. Few apply for the job. They are chosen, generally from birth or a very young age as having the potential to communicate with these spirits – puberty is a popular time to discover abilities. Initiation and training can be long, painful, even ordeal-like. This is interpreted as the spirits testing an individual's mettle, especially if they are resistant to their calling, though they may also discover guardian spirits in the form of animals. The shaman will eventually become skilled in magic,

medicine and botany, and the specific ways their community combines the three.

Shamans employ various techniques to enter an altered state of consciousness, including chant, dance, music and psychoactives derived from plants, animals or fungi. They may commune with the spirit world to diagnose ailments resistant to regular herbal medicines. A psychoactive plant rarely heals by itself; rather, it reveals the cause of the complaint. The shaman may also use visions to help someone find something lost or stolen, detect the presence of witchcraft or the evil eye, or pass through a milestone in life – from birth and adolescence and into the next world. In communities where people undertake their own vision quests, a shaman is usually present to guide them through the process.

It is easy to fall under the spell of the shaman stereotype, usually originating from the prejudices of Western organized religion and more recent forms of militant atheism. The "Hollywood shaman" is a terrifying individual, usually either an "exotic" gatekeeper for the hero, or a downright charlatan, and there are quacks who trap gullible people into buying snake oil. Genuine practitioners today, however, perform a vital role in keeping a community's spiritual knowledge and, with it, a profound history that may go back hundreds of years.

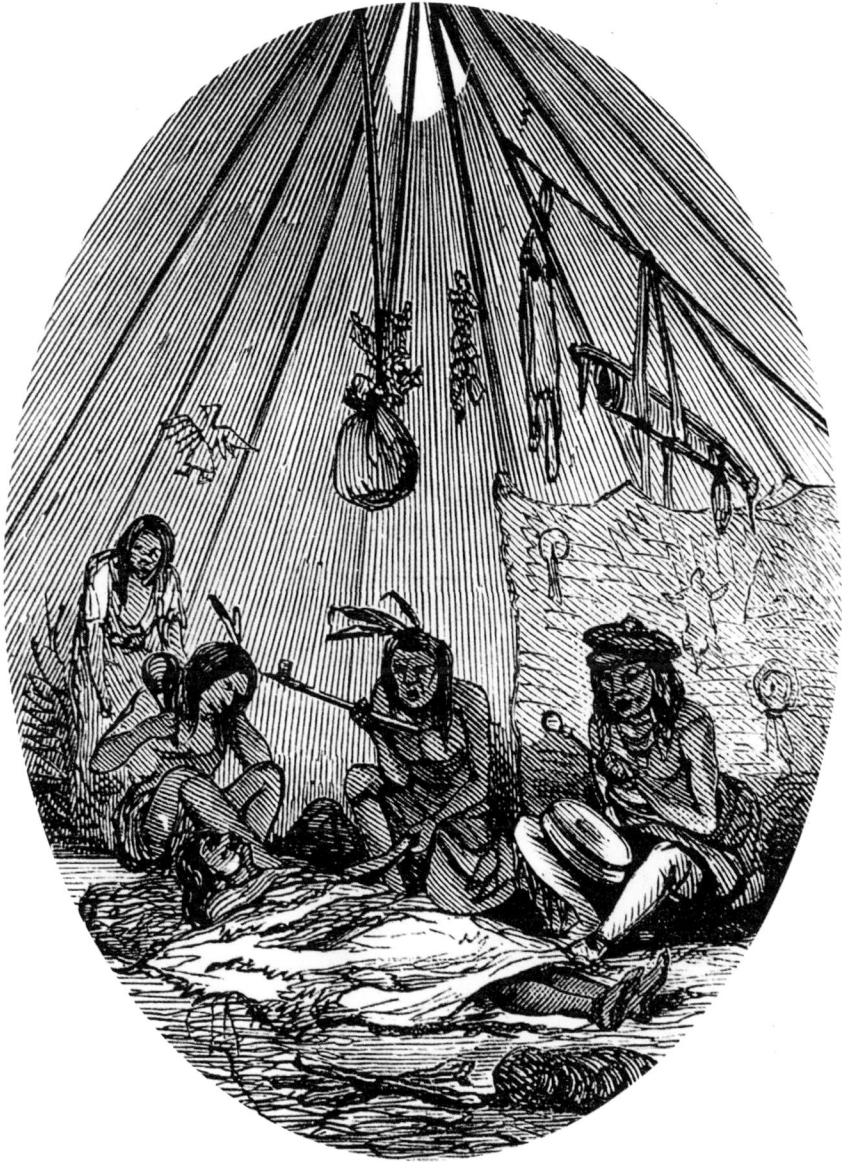

Above A sweat lodge is a ceremonial sauna and an
important event in some Native American cultures
where medicine men work on patients.

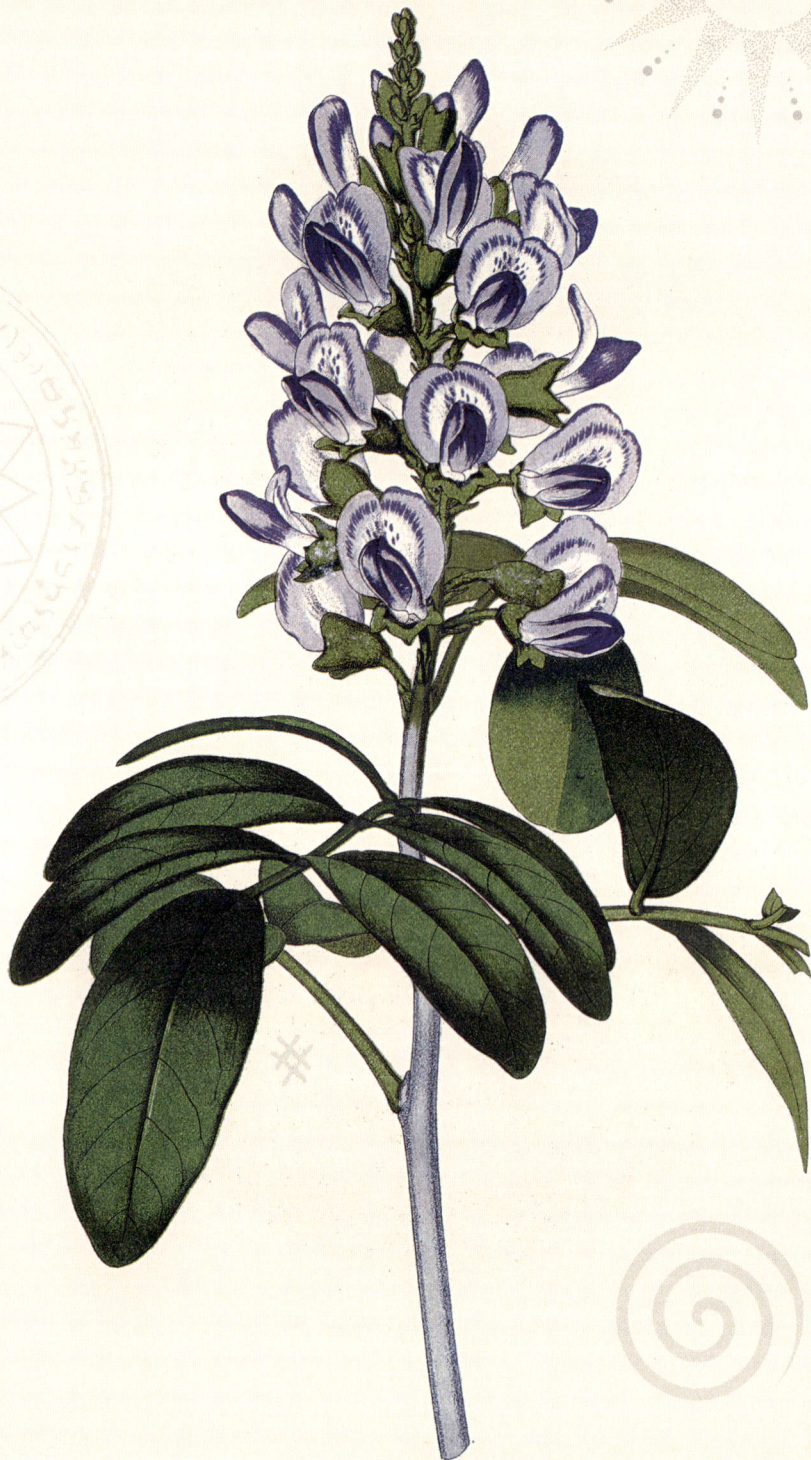

Mescal bean

Dermatophyllum secundiflorum

Native American legend tells how the trickster Coyote once made humans drunk with mescal bean so he could cut off their hair and rob them. The poor Texas mountain laurel has enjoyed a chequered reputation ever since.

A single scarlet bean from this fragrant, purple-flowered evergreen is enough to hospitalize an adult, but this did not stop several nations using it in hallucinogenic rituals and dances.

The word *mescal* is confusing. Despite being native to Texas, New Mexico and Mexico, the plant is from the pea family and does not contain mescaline like the peyote cactus also found there (see p. 180). Its alkaloid, cytisine, more closely resembles nicotine. Mescal bean is also entirely unrelated to the agave used in the alcoholic drink mezcal.

When dried, mescal bean's pods make excellent rattles, while individual beans may be threaded like beads. Beans found in rock shelters may date as far back as 6,500 years and archaeologists have found mescal-decorated buckskin loincloths, cradleboards and even a small "healer's kit" containing the beans alongside tools, sinew and jackrabbit jaws. The Comanche used mescal bean for earaches, the Cheyenne as an eyewash.

The nineteenth century was a difficult time for the indigenous people of America. As colonists raided their lands and destroyed their communities, at least a dozen nations created secret mescal bean cults dedicated to keeping their traditions alive. The plant's blood-red seeds were sewn onto warriors' clothing: shirts, leggings, necklaces, headdresses and bandoliers.

In ritual, the beans were usually roasted, then chewed or swallowed. This would induce staggering, intoxication, convulsions, the evacuation of both stomach and bowels, paralysis, "seeing red", increased heart rate and, presumably, not a few accidental deaths. Its use may also encourage imaginary visions.

Perhaps understandably, accounts are vague. One Lenape who attended an Apache ceremony described participants jumping out of the tipi's smoke hole, before coming back in through the entrance and walking barefoot across live coals. One particularly hardcore Pawnee Deer Dance required initiates to consume the mixture until they fell unconscious. This was tested by scraping the spiked teeth of garfish up the new member's spine. One flinch and he was out.

Although mescal bean still has resonance among several nations, especially Comanche, it has largely given way to peyote in ritual use, probably because it is so very dangerous.

Egyptian lotus

Nymphaea caerulea
var. *caerulea*

One of the most beautiful sculptures of the ancient world depicts the young Pharaoh Tutankhamun in the guise of Nefertem, Waterlily of the Sun, his painted wooden head emerging from a lotus flower.

Nefertem rose from the primal waters as a blue lotus, but by Tutankhamun's time he was usually represented as a beautiful youth surrounded by waterlily flowers. *Nymphaea caerulea* var. *caerulea* opens with the dawn, follows the daylight and then closes at dusk, making it an important symbol of Ra, the Sun god. It also represents life, blossoming at birth and fading on entering the darkness of the underworld, presided over by Osiris, who also claims the plant. Both the ancient Egyptian and Mayan cultures used it for purification rituals.

Some *Nymphaea* contain the alkaloid nuciferine, rendering them at best inedible, though the rhizomes of some species, with careful preparation, have been eaten. The blue lotus is one of these; its starchy "roots" are boiled or roasted, but rarely relished. Other alkaloids in *N. caerulea* var. *caerulea* are still being investigated, with some studies suggesting it may contain apomorphine. Scientists are currently examining the possibilities of apomorphine's dopamine receptor binding qualities to alleviate Parkinson's disease symptoms. Blue lotus's mild sedative effect may be responsible for its reputation as a dream-enhancer, the apomorphine and nuciferine considered partly responsible for various reports of lucid dreaming. Limited data is available on the safety of the blue lotus for human consumption.

Lotus has enjoyed another intriguing reputation since antiquity: as an aphrodisiac. One notorious document, the Turin Papyrus, even features it in erotic cartoons. Recent research revealed that apomorphine could be of interest to treat erectile dysfunction. Perhaps the ancients knew this all along, though Pliny the Elder, always the contrarian, pronounced lotus as an antidote to love potions. He even claimed that drinking crushed waterlily in vinegar for 10 days will turn a boy into a eunuch.

The waterlily has always presented a powerful image. An ancient Syrian plaque shows the mysterious goddess Asherah holding a lotus blossom, while several Mayan archaeological sites have revealed lotus-themed artefacts. A Native American legend tells how a star fell to earth, and on landing in a lake, turned into a flower. For Buddhists, lotus is one of the eight auspicious symbols, representing the victory over self. Both the Buddha and the Hindu god Shiva are often shown in the Padmasana or lotus position, a cross-legged meditation pose also used in Tantric and Jain contemplation.

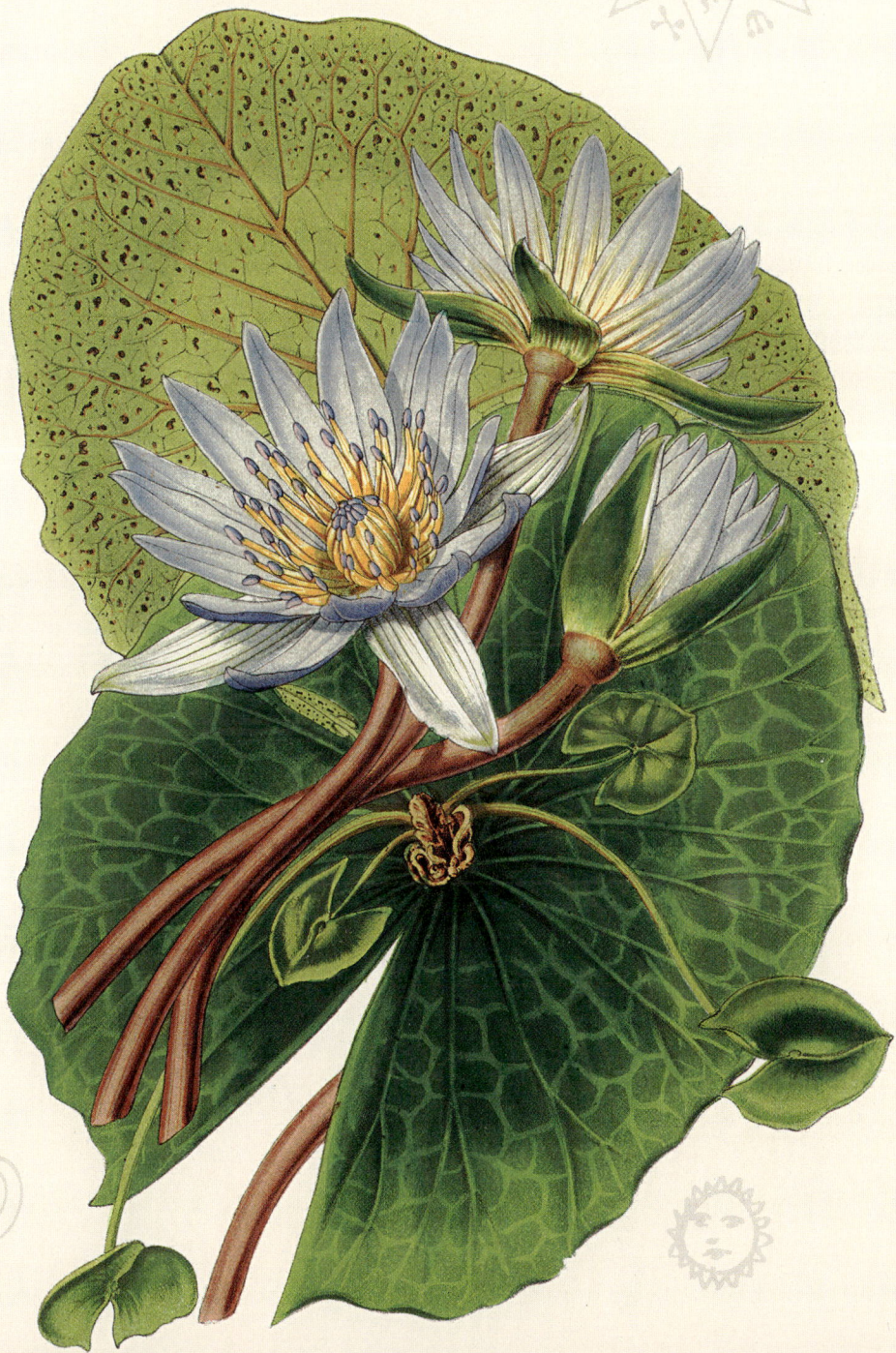

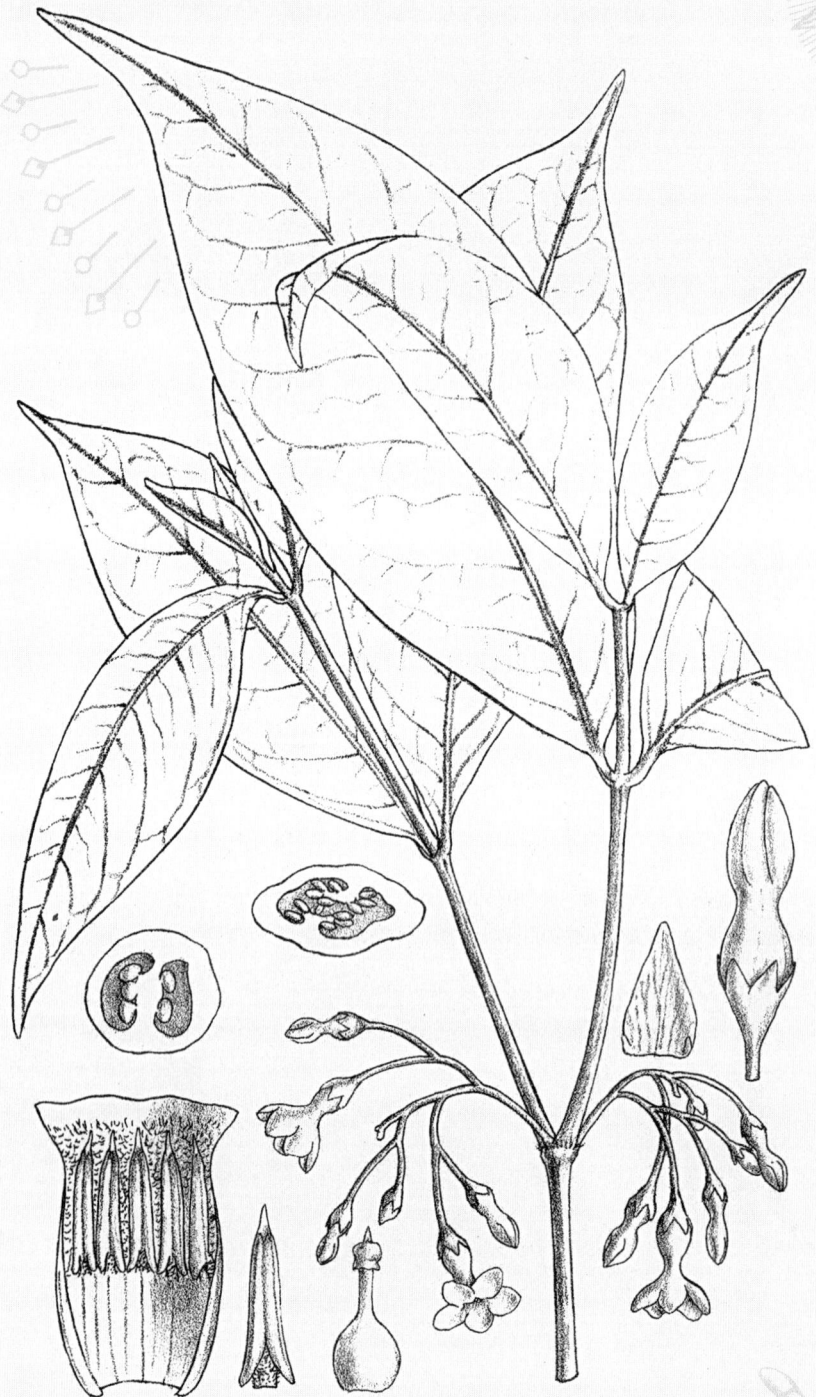

Iboga

Tabernanthe iboga

Mebege the Creator god was alone in the universe with only
Dibobia the spider for company, so he made an egg from
strands of his hair, a piece of his brain and a smooth stone.
Dibobia threw the egg into the ocean.

Three deities were born, the greatest of which was Zame ye Mebege, god of the Sun. Zame ye Mebege spotted a human called Bitam, picking the fruit of the Atanga tree, and caused Bitam to fall and die, then cut off his fingers and toes and planted them. Wherever the digits fell, an iboga bush sprouted.

Many of the rainforest-dwelling people of West Africa, and in particular Gabon, practise Bwiti, a spiritual discipline based around the hallucinogenic properties of iboga. An evergreen shrub from the dogbane family, *Tabernanthe iboga* produces delicate pink and white flowers and curious orange fruit, but these are generally overlooked for the yellowy-brown bark of the plant's roots. Usually ground into a powder, this tough outer casing becomes a powerful psychoactive substance that Bwiti followers, usually from Fang, Mitsogo and Punu communities, consume to commune with their ancestors.

Iboga contains a complex cocktail of alkaloids including ibogaine, which can affect the body's neurotransmitters such as serotonin and dopamine. Ibogaine is a hallucinogen. In small doses it is a stimulant, considered to enable hunters and travellers to stay awake longer and carry heavier loads. Larger doses can result in vivid hallucinations, vomiting, convulsions, loss of motor function, paralysis, respiratory seizure and temporary unconsciousness. An overdose may result in death.

Iboga has been used by women and it is obligatory for men to undergo an initiation rite to join the Bwiti faith. This involves consuming large quantities of iboga, guided by a Nganga (spiritual leader), to become a *baanzi*: someone who has "broken open their head" and seen the other world with their own eyes. Afterwards it is believed they will be able to consume iboga on a regular basis as medicine, to diagnose illness, to honour the ancestors, drive out evil spirits and for personal development.

The initiation is not undergone lightly. Most participants will collapse at some point; a very few will remain permanently in the other world. Men and women undergo similar rites, but separately in segregated spaces. Some paint themselves white and dress in raffia skirts decorated with shells or beads. Music, including rattles, drums and the *mongongo*, a bow-harp played with the mouth, accompanies singing and dancing, sometimes lit by a traditional torch called a *mupeto*, made from bark and tree sap. The ceremony begins at night and can last from three to seven days.

With large doses, the first sense affected is usually hearing, leading to nausea, vomiting, disorientation and extreme dizziness. Photosensitivity can also occur. The initiate is lain down and watched as they witness between three and six hours of surreal waking dreams, commonly including memories and images of the past, which may help to account for Bwiti's focus on ancestors. Accounts of encounters with spirits often reflect harrowing experiences. A much longer secondary phase heralds up to 10 hours of personal introspection, where the user examines their inner thoughts. Even after this, residual stimulation may last for weeks.

In 1962 American heroin addict Howard Lotsof took iboga while searching for a stronger high, but after consumption, discovered he had no further desire for drugs. After decades of research as to whether it may somehow "reset" the brain, the jury is still out on iboga's potential as an anti-addiction treatment, since its side effects can be extremely hazardous and even lethal. While there do seem to be incidental reports of people discontinuing addictive habits, if someone takes a normal dose of their addicted drug after an iboga trip, they may run an increased risk of overdosing.

Conducting research has been made even more difficult since iboga has been banned in many countries, but the current opioid epidemic has seen a rise in people desperate to curb their addiction and willing to take the risk, aware that they may die from an overdose anyway. There is currently a boom in clinics – in the countries that have not proscribed the drug – offering ibogaine as a part of drug rehabilitation. Some are fully accredited medical facilities, others are not, and the ethics of using ibogaine as therapy are still in their infancy, with strong feelings on all sides. As the drug gains interest outside Africa, poachers are stripping the rainforest of the wild plant and selling the herb (and any number of fakes) on the black market.

Iboga remains extremely popular in the Gabonese Republic, where Bwiti is one of the three official religions, despite its being denounced by one of the others, the Catholic Church. In 2000, the plant was declared a Gabonese National Treasure.

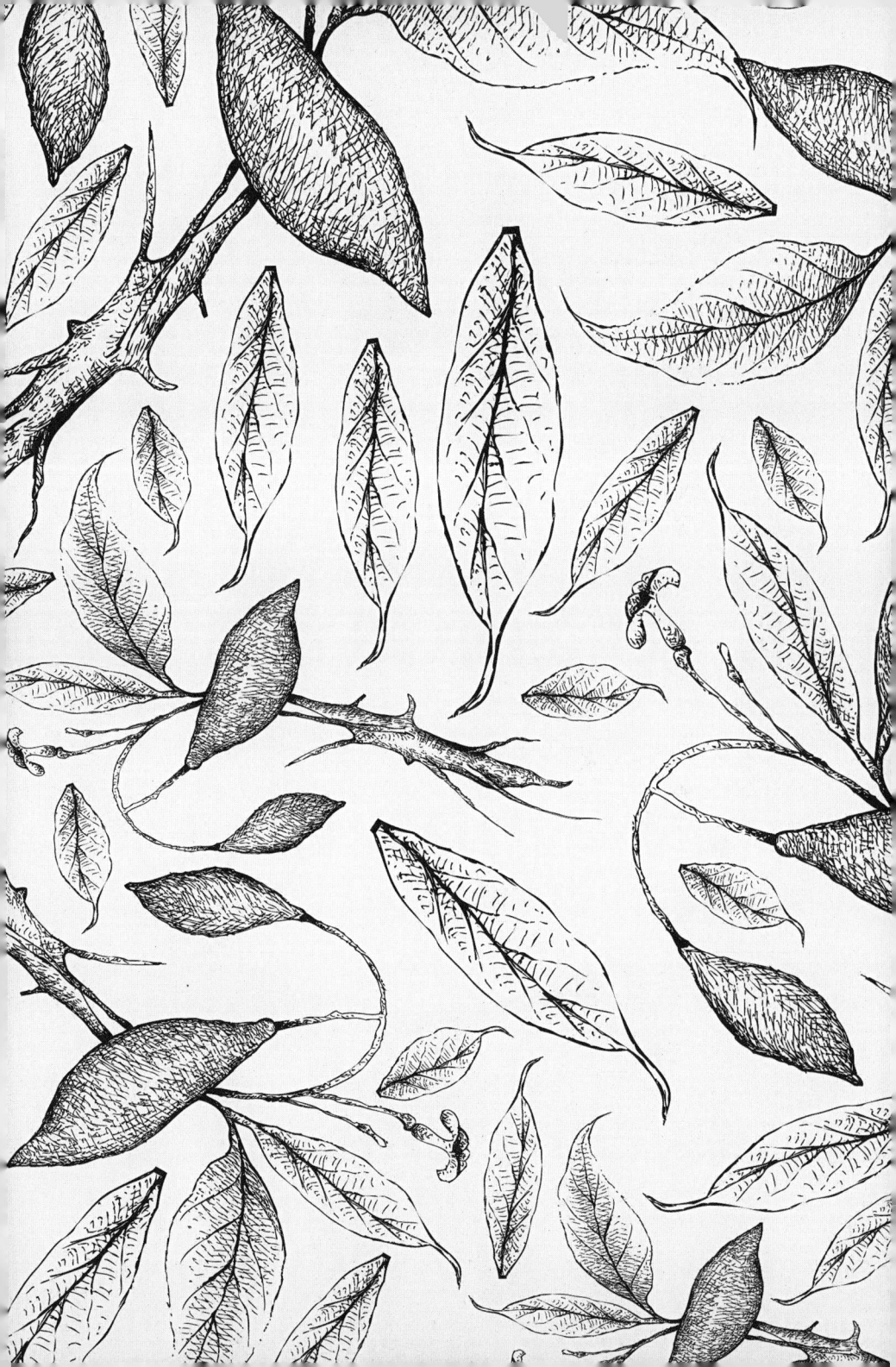

Chapter 2:

Home Comforts (Everyday stimulants)

Coffee. Tea. Chocolate. There can be few people – in the Western world, at least – who do not enjoy at least one of these deliciously quotidian "home comforts" on a daily basis. While some of the substances in this book seem exotic, even dangerous, such everyday stimulants are so omnipresent it rarely occurs to us that all three carry psychoactive effects of one kind or another. And that's before we add a little sweetness to the mix…

Life's Little Pick-Me-Ups

Caffeine is the most widely used legal stimulant on the planet.
We consume around 100,000 tonnes of it each year, mainly
in the form of tea, coffee and chocolate.

Most Europeans had never experienced it until the sixteenth century, but they soon caught up...

Caffeine is a plant's insecticide, protecting its most vulnerable parts, including coffee beans, tea leaves and cocoa beans. Perhaps ironically, this makes those parts perfect targets for the plant's most dangerous predators: us. A neurotransmitter in our bodies that helps us sleep is counteracted by caffeine, making us more alert and giving us the energy to face the day. It also promotes concentration, though taken too far it may overstimulate us into heart palpitations, diarrhoea and insomnia. We can also develop a caffeine dependency, though not all scientists agree it is a classically addictive drug because the reward it offers the brain is not large enough to unbalance the system in the same way as drugs such as amphetamines and cocaine.

Many see that slight headache until the first fix of the day as a side effect of so many other, better reactions. Coffee is the student's friend, enabling those overnighter essay-writing marathons. The first thing every British person will do on the arrival of bad news of any variety is make a pot of tea, while the now traditional solace of jilted lovers is the largest bar of chocolate they can find.

There are around 131 species of *Coffea*, three of which are commercially grown. Arabica (*C. arabica*) is considered to have the finest flavour; robusta (*C. canephora*) is coarser but cheaper. Liberica (*C. liberica*) counts for only around 2% of the world's production but, as climate change and deforestation threaten supplies of robusta and arabica, may come into its own yet.

Cocoa (probably a misspelling of cacao) made its way to Europe in the sixteenth century, by now sweetened with sugar and flavoured with spices. By the seventeenth century the drink, served in rowdy "chocolate houses" from Vienna to London, was as popular – and as stimulating – as coffee and tea.

While each stimulant has its own history, legends and mythology, general caffeine folklore is equally everyday, often stemming from personal rituals, perhaps to start the day, or in a special way of brewing a pot of tea. Until rationing in the Second World War, for example, the "correct" teamaking method included one spoonful of leaves for each person and one "for the pot". Small rituals turn, over the years, into superstitions. Does stirring your coffee with a fork really foment trouble for the day? Might stirring tea anticlockwise do the same? Who knows, but for some people such fancies become as ingrained as avoiding black cats and ladders.

Opposite During the London Blitz, hot cups of tea were served on mobile canteens around the city.

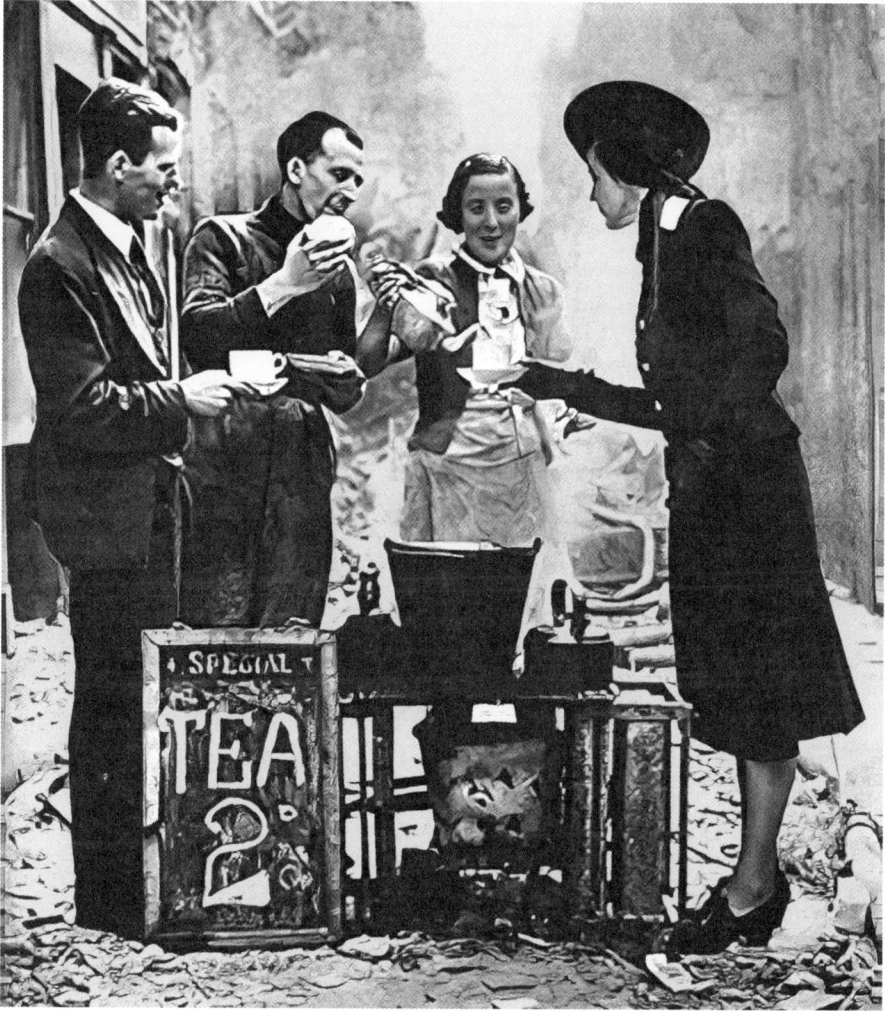

Tasseomancy (aka *tasseography*) is the art of interpreting the shapes left by tea leaves or coffee grounds in the bottom of the cup, though its origins lie in divination via wine sediments. Usually associated with Romani people, the practice spread throughout Europe, using whichever drink was most popular in a country, only slightly behind crystal balls and palm-reading in popularity. During Victorian times, "reading the leaves" became a party game, involving special books and even chinaware, printed with the meanings of strange formations found in the bottom of an empty cup.

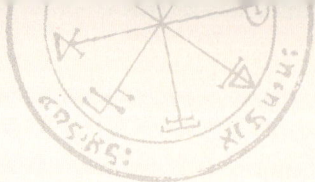

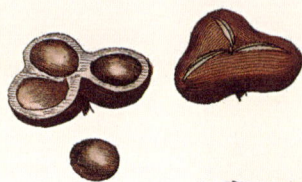

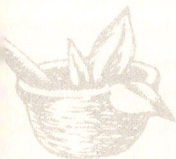

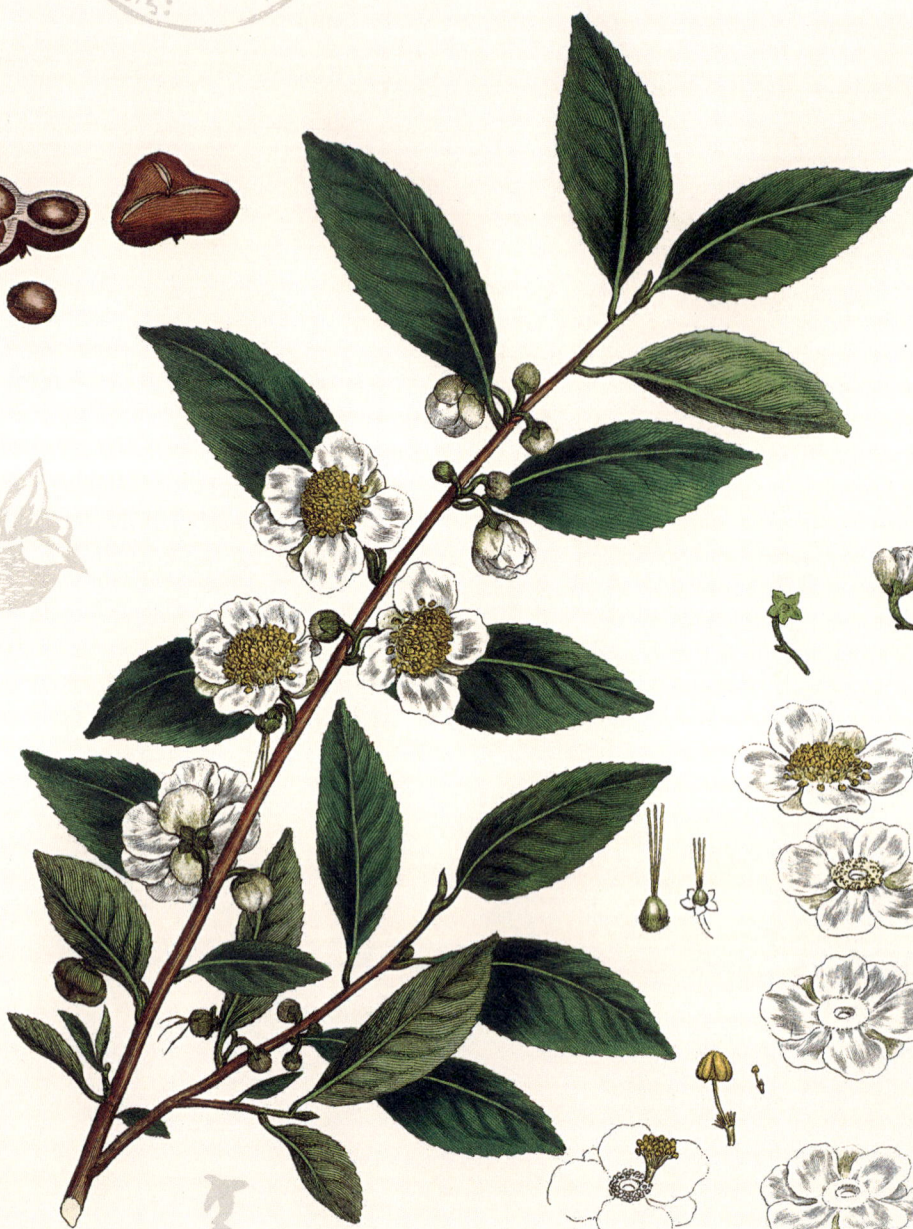

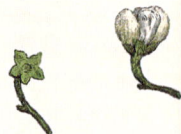

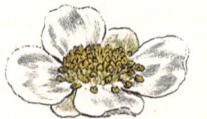

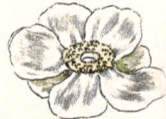

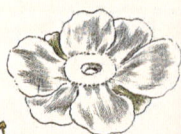

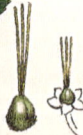

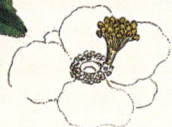

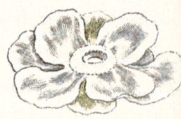

Tea

Camellia sinensis

In 2737 BCE, Shennong, the legendary emperor and farmer,
was boiling water in his garden. A leaf (perhaps three) floated
from a nearby tree into his pot and tea was invented.

Precise dates, when dealing with events that happened more than 4,000 years ago, are usually a bit of a folklore red flag, especially when dealing with mythical figures. On the other hand, that is what folklore is – legends, tales, myths – and whether or not they are true, it's the stories that count. Should we be any more convinced by the tree that grew from the Zen Buddhist monk Bodhidharma's eyelids, which he cut off to stay awake while meditating? It is said he then brewed leaves from the tree to make a refreshing drink. Certainly, tea has been China's national drink since the Tang Dynasty (618–907), associated with Buddhist, Taoist and Confucian traditions.

Legend also tells us that Lu Yu (733–804) was an orphan adopted into the Dragon Cloud Monastery, but would not take the robe and ran away to become a circus clown. A local governor spotted the 14-year-old and offered to help him study. The boy found purpose in tea, writing in his monograph *Chájīng* (*The Classic of Tea*) that the brew symbolized balance and harmony within the universe. His almost contemporary, Lu Tong (790–835), wrote *Seven Bowls of Tea*, a poem that guides the reader through the mind-altering stages of drinking the brew while meditating. After moistening his lips with the first

bowl and breaking his loneliness with the second, Lu Tong enters his own body to find the five thousand scrolls of the mind. By the fourth bowl he is beginning to perspire as evil leaves him; a fifth purifies his bones, while a sixth calls him to Penglai, land of the immortals. He does not even need to drink the seventh bowl: he has transcended to a higher level. *The Cha Dao* tea ceremony still follows Lu Tong's principles of balance.

The thirteenth-century explorer Marco Polo discussed tea in his travel writings, but the drink did not catch on in the West until the seventeenth century. It was particularly embraced by women, who were not allowed in the coffee houses. Taking a "dish" of tea developed into a genteel fashion, but China understandably kept the secrets of growing *Camellia sinensis* and tea was an expensive pastime. Adding to a very long list of dodgy dealings, the British East India Company sent botanist Robert Fortune into the heartlands, disguised as a Chinese merchant. Fortune learned tea's farming techniques, and sneaked samples back to the East India Company, who promptly established plantations in India, later joined by local Assam variety *C. sinensis* var. *assamica*. Prices tumbled, and tea became available to all.

Across the Atlantic, tea had originally been introduced by the Dutch, but the British East India Company (yes, again...) convinced Parliament to impose heavy taxes on the now-British colony. Unsurprisingly, Americans were unhappy and, in 1773, a number of other grievances collided with the new Tea Act, resulting in the notorious Boston Tea Party, where protesters disguised as Native Americans dumped an entire shipment into Boston Harbour. This didn't stop American fondness for the beverage, experimenting with iced versions and the first commercial tea bags. Cocking a small snook to the British, "English Breakfast Tea" was first mentioned in 1843 by New York tea merchant Richard Davies who, admittedly, sold it as being all the rage in England. We do not know what was in Davies's blend, but by 1892 Queen Victoria was drinking a tea of the same name at Balmoral, Scotland. Today, the robust blend of Assam, Ceylon and Kenyan teas is drunk all day long by British folk— and is what you get if you fail to specify what kind of tea you're ordering.

The way we drink tea may have changed over the years, but its transformative properties remain. The first thing many Brits will do in the event of any tragedy is to put the kettle on; whether expensive "living tea" or supermarket teabags, the results – at once calming and stimulating – allow us to keep calm and carry on.

During the Second World War, food rationing saw tea reduced to two ounces per person per week. This did not stop it becoming a symbol of national unity on the Home Front. One of the war's most famous images depicts a woman sitting on top of rubble after an air raid, sipping a cuppa. On the actual Front, every Centurion tank was equipped with a BV (boiling vessel), part number FV706656. The most junior member of the team was designated "BV Commander", with essential tea making duties. British tanks still include them, retaining the same serial number, though they are now designated "cooking vessels" (CV). When tea became one of the first goods to come off rationing in 1952, it was front-page news.

There are any number of superstitions accompanying tea. Leaving your spoon upside down invites bad news, while bad luck inevitably follows a broken teapot. Putting tea leaves on the fire, however, will ward off poverty. It is worth a punt – for being unable to afford a cup of tea is, surely, the worst luck of all.

Opposite Tea is always a good idea: women enjoying a tea party in 1899.

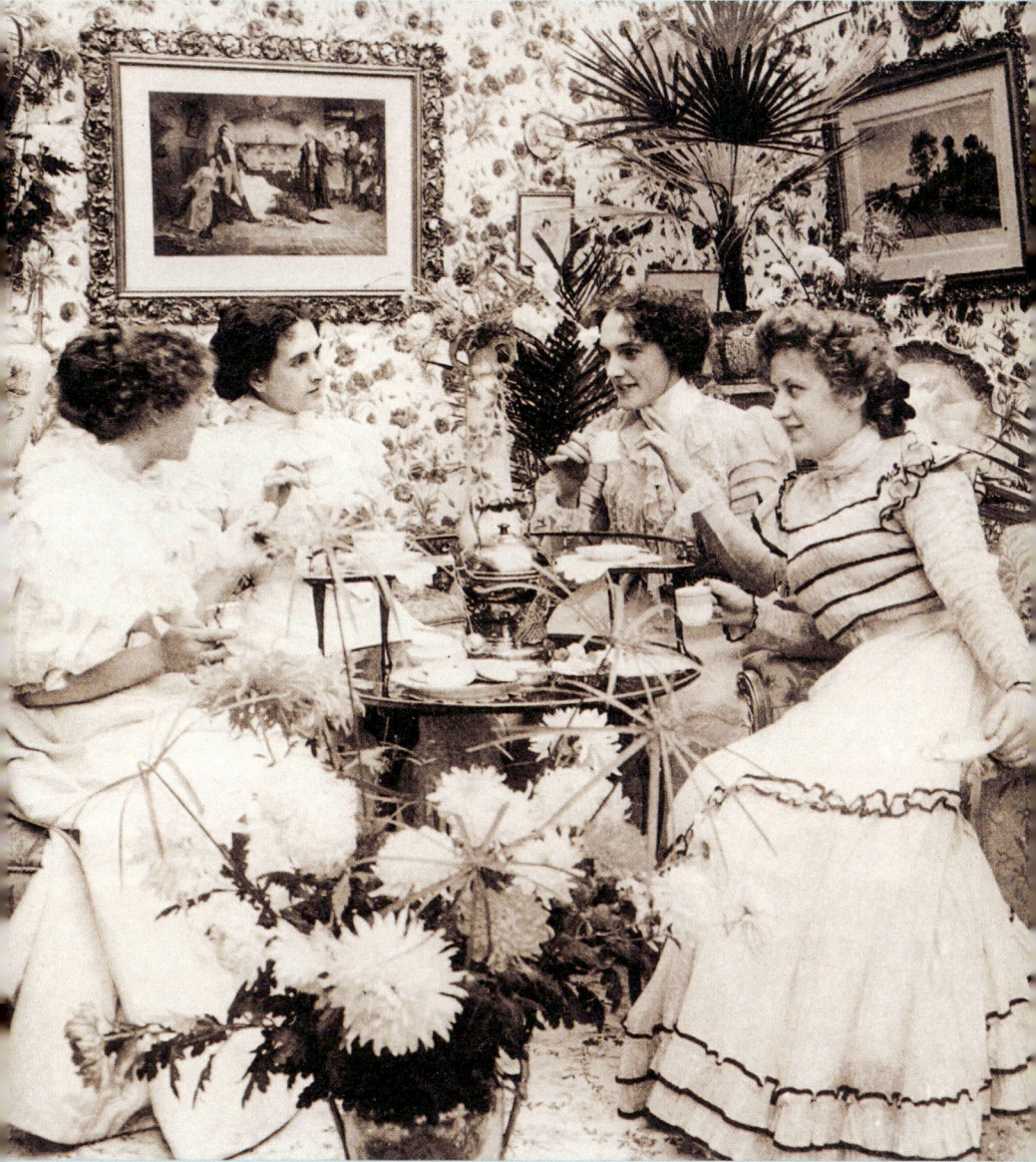

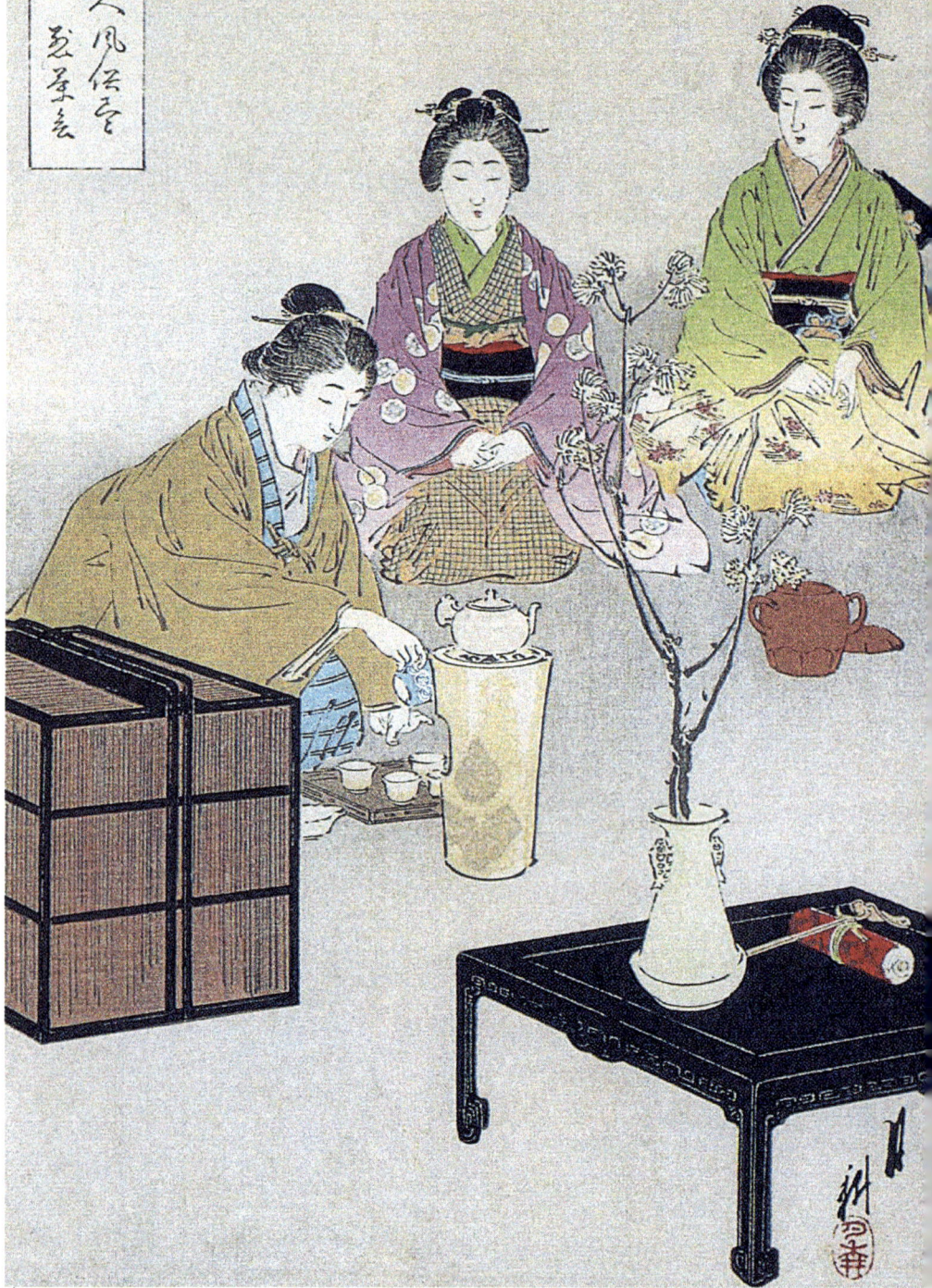

The Way of Tea

Wabi-sabi is a philosophy based on the acceptance of life as fragile, imperfect and transient. Taking time to appreciate such beauty and vulnerability is the secret of happiness.

The art of *chanoyu* – way of tea – is uniquely Japanese, even though both tea and the Zen Buddhist principles behind its serving originated in China. Every aspect of the ritual is heavy with symbolism.

While the rest of the world (and, indeed, the Japanese, in their daily lives) infuse dried tea leaves for their daily cuppa, chanoyu uses matcha, a green, powdered form, formally whipped with boiled water using a bamboo *chasen* (whisk). The resulting frothy, bitter-tasting brew is served in hand-crafted *chawan* (tea bowls). The amount of caffeine in matcha varies, but it is rarely strong. No one becomes intoxicated. The ceremony is cerebral, but it is the event that affects the mind, not chemicals.

Tea was introduced to Japan in the 700s, but it was the thirteenth-century Zen Buddhist monk Eisai who brought matcha – and its preparation – back from China. The ceremony was codified in the sixteenth century by the great master Sen Rikyū, who championed simplicity above everything, using exquisite equipment selected for its beauty.

Chanoyu embodies four principles: harmony, respect, purity and tranquillity. It takes place either in a *chashitsu* (tea cabin), originally within formal gardens, or a dedicated room. A typical chashitsu is the size of four and a half tatami mats (7.4m², 77sq ft); many are much smaller, celebrating intimacy. Sliding translucent doors may be supplemented with another, low entrance, forcing guests to crawl inside, a symbol of humility. A *tokonoma* (alcove) contains a seasonally appropriate scroll and/or flower arrangement. A sunken fireplace boils the kettle in winter; in summer a small brazier suffices.

Guests wash, formally greet their host, then sit in silence as the tea is prepared. This may take several hours, including a multi-course *kaiseki* meal and thick tea before the thinner variety, though today's ceremonies are generally shorter.

Using minimal, precise movements, the host places the bowl in front of their guest, who lifts it with both hands, rotating it so the decorative front faces outwards. The tea is sipped and appreciated, the bowl wiped with thumb and forefinger, rotated once more then returned to the mat. Only then will the company speak, usually of the choices of utensils employed that day. The host themself does not drink.

Tea is ingrained at every level of Japanese society, and perfecting its serving is part of basic geisha (entertainer) training. *Ochaya*, where geisha live and work from, literally means *tea house*. Once common countrywide, the term is now used exclusively for establishments in Kyoto. Tea, however, remains universal.

Opposite Tea is ingrained in Japanese culture. This illustration from 1888 depicts a traditional Japanese Tea Ceremony.

Coffee

Coffea arabica

Ethiopian legend tells how a goatherd named Kaldi noticed his animals eating berries from a certain tree and becoming so excitable they would not settle at night.

On consulting the abbot of a local monastery, he learned the monks made a drink with the fruit to stay awake during hours of prayer. Coffee had been born. Human use of the "cherries" from wild *Coffea* trees probably originated in sixth-century Ethiopia. The drink reached Yemen by about 1100, though of course it has its own origin story there, too, where a man named Omar was exiled into the hills. Starving, he found some red berries, whose kernels he roasted, then boiled. He drank the cooking water, instantly reviving his spirits. News spread quickly, and "Omar the Healer" and his magic beverage were welcomed back to the port of Mocha.

In Turkey, where coffee is celebrated as a UNESCO element of intangible cultural heritage, every part of production and consumption is swathed in ritual. Served in tiny cups, the strong brew represents hospitality, refinement and friendship, especially at traditional ceremonies and holidays. Some use the grounds to tell fortunes.

The first English coffee house was opened in Oxford in 1650; two years later another opened in

Opposite An advert for Van Ysendyk coffee, a Belgian coffee brand advertised in the 1930s with art deco posters like this one.

St Michael's Alley in the City of London. The famous insurance market Lloyds of London began as a coffee shop in 1668, but the beverage was not just for men of finance (and it was just men; the only women allowed inside such establishments were sex-workers). Intellectuals also met in coffee houses, including some who wanted more than a caffeine hit. The 1789 French Revolution fomented in coffee houses, as did a whole slew of insurgencies during 1848, the Year of Revolution.

Every country has its coffee traditions and methods, from the espressos of Vienna swathed with whipped cream, through battered enamel jugs boiled over campfires by America's pioneers, to Italy where, in 1933, Luigi di Ponti sold the patent to his stovetop "moka pot" to Alfonso Bialetti, spawning a modern classic.

Coffee remains a popular drink in Arabic countries, which often have strict rules against alcohol, but until recently many Africans avoided it. Aggressive world commodities markets reminded them of an unpleasant colonial past. Increasingly, however, as farmers regain control of production, African people are rediscovering the drink their ancestors enjoyed.

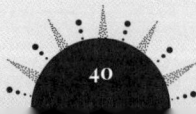

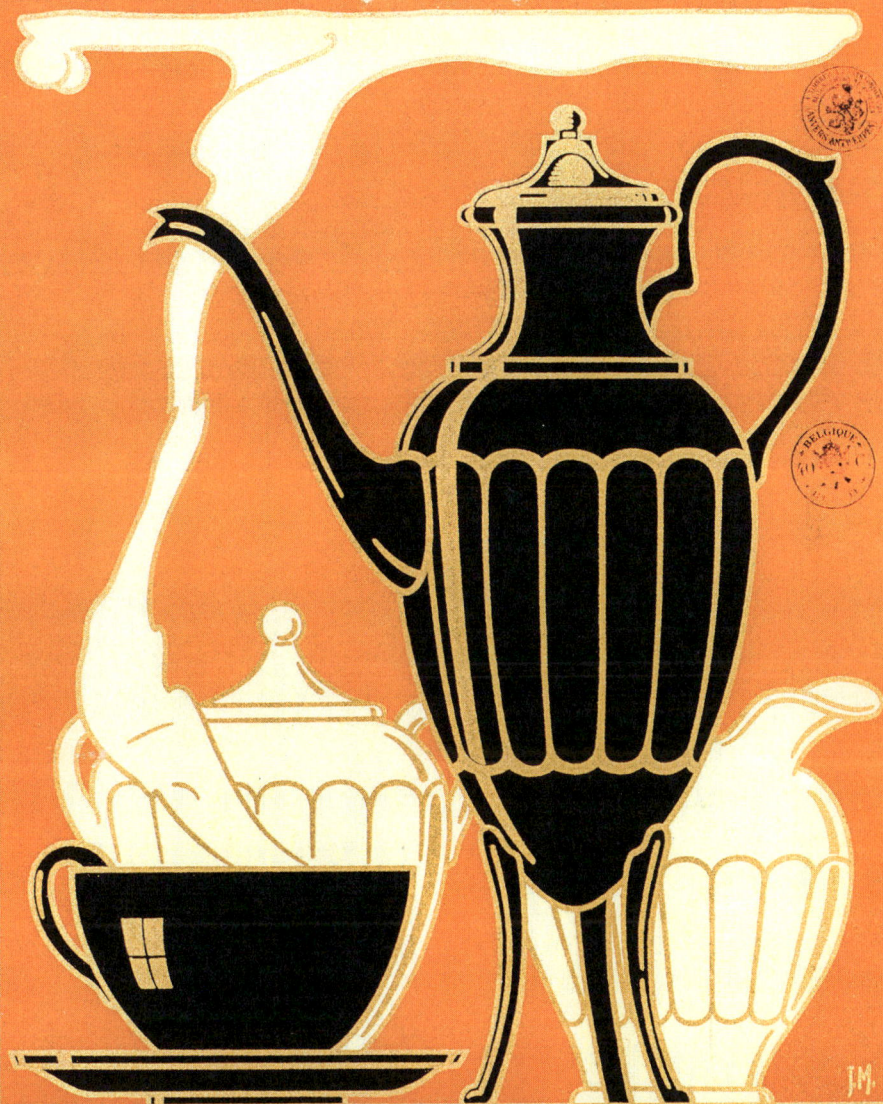

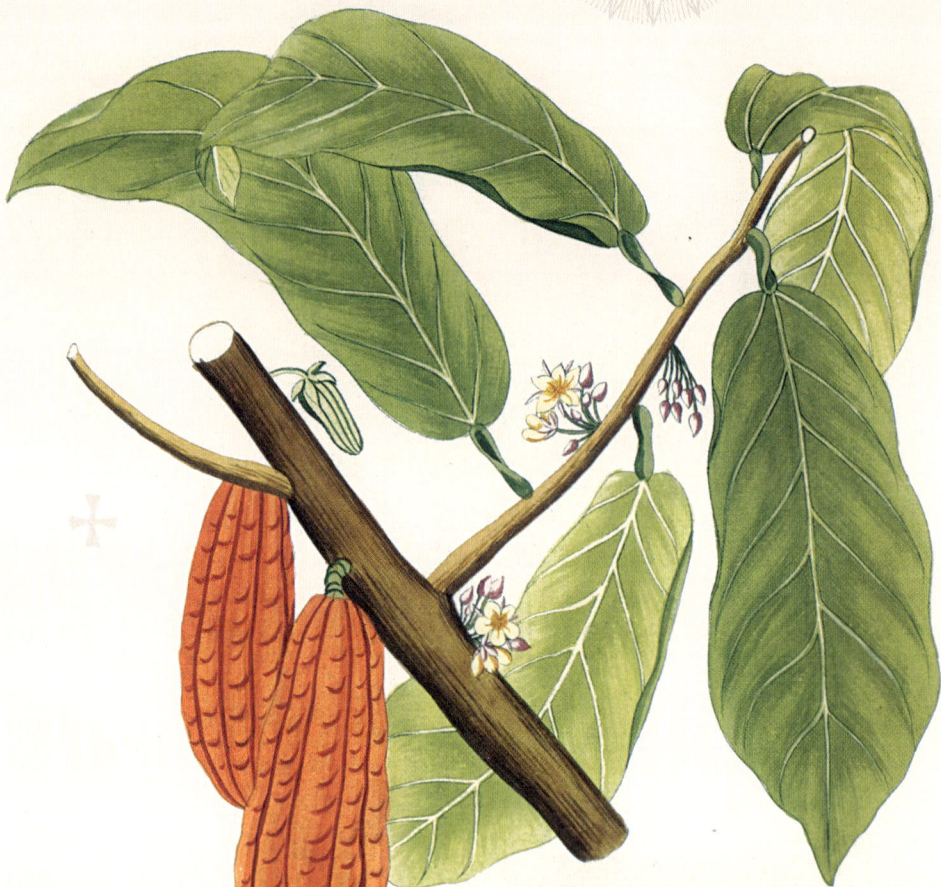

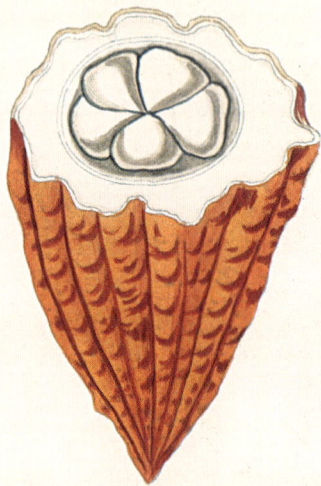

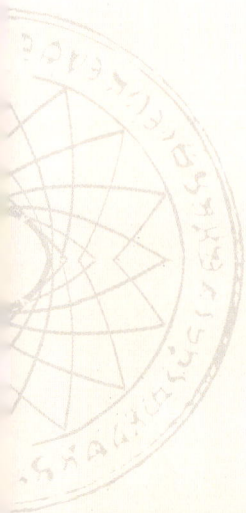

Cocoa

Theobroma cacao

It seems that half the world describes itself as "chocoholic" these days, unable to resist the sticky delights of the bean that Carl Linnaeus, the father of modern taxonomy, called *Theobroma*, "food of the gods". They would be half-right.

Cocoa is not considered to be addictive, but we might be forgiven for assuming it is, thanks to psychoactive agents called methylxanthines, such as theobromine, which may influence our mood and alertness. Theobromine helps blood vessels relax and widen, which may help lower blood pressure. Another compound, phenylethylamine, may raise blood pressure and heighten sensations in a similar way to the chemical messengers produced in the brain when someone falls in love.

The people who lived in Santa Ana (La Florida), in modern-day Ecuador, around 3500 BCE did not know any such science, of course, but they enjoyed the effects. They domesticated the cacao tree, though it was probably the Olmecs of southern Mexico who first roasted and ground the beans to drink. Mayan mythology tells us humans were created when the gods mixed divine blood with *kakaw*. A step pyramid in the Mayan city of Palanque even has a carving that depicts the seventh-century queen Sak K'uk reborn as a cacao tree.

Cacao is most closely associated with the Aztecs. As an empire, they could demand tributes in the form of beans, which were transformed into a frothy drink called *xocolatl* ("bitter water"). They told stories of how Quetzacoatl, the feathered serpent god of light, brought the cacao tree from a sacred mountain, gave it to their predecessors the Toltecs and taught their women how to make the drink.

Xocolatl sealed diplomatic alliances, business deals and marriages. It was drunk at religious rituals and bound sacrificial victims to their fates. It was used as a medicine, digestif and reward to warriors, but it was not consumed universally. The cold, bitter beverage was reserved mainly for gods and royalty. The emperor Moctezuma II habitually drank *xocolatl* from a golden cup before visiting his many wives. Rather more disastrously he gave some to the conquistador Hernán Cortés.

The Spanish invaders were not initially impressed with cacao, but missionaries encouraged their indigenous converts to offer beans to Christian icons instead of their old gods, resulting in peculiar blends of religious imagery. El Señor del Cacao (The Lord of Chocolate), in Mexico City, is the world's only statue of Christ dedicated to chocolate.

Sugarcane

Saccharum officinarum

While it can produce great feelings of satisfaction and energy, sugar is not a classic hallucinogen. Yet it is a classic stimulant and studies on rodents suggest it may be highly addictive.

Such research is controversial, with opponents claiming sugar is merely habit-forming rather than addictive, but most agree that "glucose signalling" has a mild psychoactive effect. The brain suddenly receives a plentiful supply of energy and begins to operate at full speed, causing a sugar rush, but this does not last long, resulting in an all-too-familiar "crash" afterwards. Anecdotally, many people report sugar cravings as intense as any desire for caffeine or nicotine, even for sex or food.

We are born with a sweet tooth. Sugars were once hard to come by, mainly found in fruits and honey. The first "sugar" seems to have been refined from *Saccharum officinarum* in India, around 2,500 years ago.

Sugar is usually portrayed as a good thing within folklore. Its mood-altering effects are touchingly portrayed in a Philippine legend, where a *datu* (chieftain) who had lost his zest for life, prayed to Bathala the creator to end it. He was told that his time on Earth was not yet done. Disappointed, he retreated to the forest, where an old man led him to a grove of sugarcane – heaven on earth – and the *datu* was able to rediscover sweetness in his world.

In India, Kama, the handsome Hindu god of erotic love and sensual pleasure, carries a bow of sugarcane. With a string of a row of bees, it shoots flowers directly into the human heart. Four-armed Tripura Sundari, one of the 10 Shakta Mahavidyas (manifestations of the supreme goddess Mahadevi), also carries such a bow, representing the mind, and five arrows, one for each of the senses.

Sugar has had a less joyful modern history, as one of the major commodities in the notorious triangular trade operating between various European powers, Africa and the Americas between the sixteenth and nineteenth centuries. *Saccharum officinarum* arrived in the West Indies in 1493 to be grown by an enslaved workforce for cheap refined sugar.

Rum was an interesting by-product, distilled from leftover sugar juice, enjoyed by the enslaved people who made it, denounced by Europeans as "rumbullion", "kill-devil" and "a hot, hellish and terrible liquor". It was not the first sugar spirit – ancient Egypt, India, Persia and Sumeria had all experimented – but it was the people's drink, which they gave to one of the gods they brought with them. Ogun or, in Haitian Vodou, Ogou, still presides over rum and rum-making today.

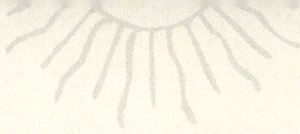

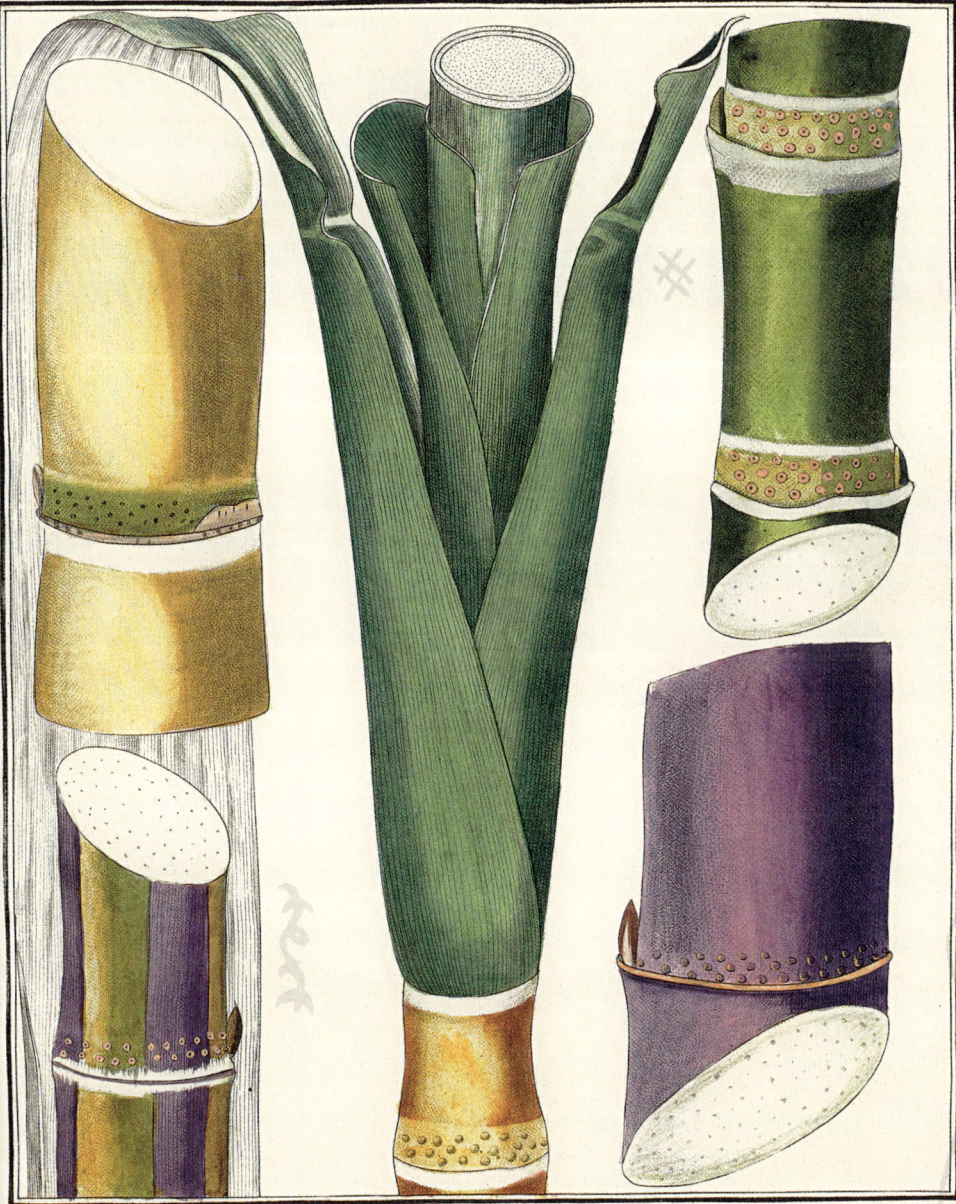

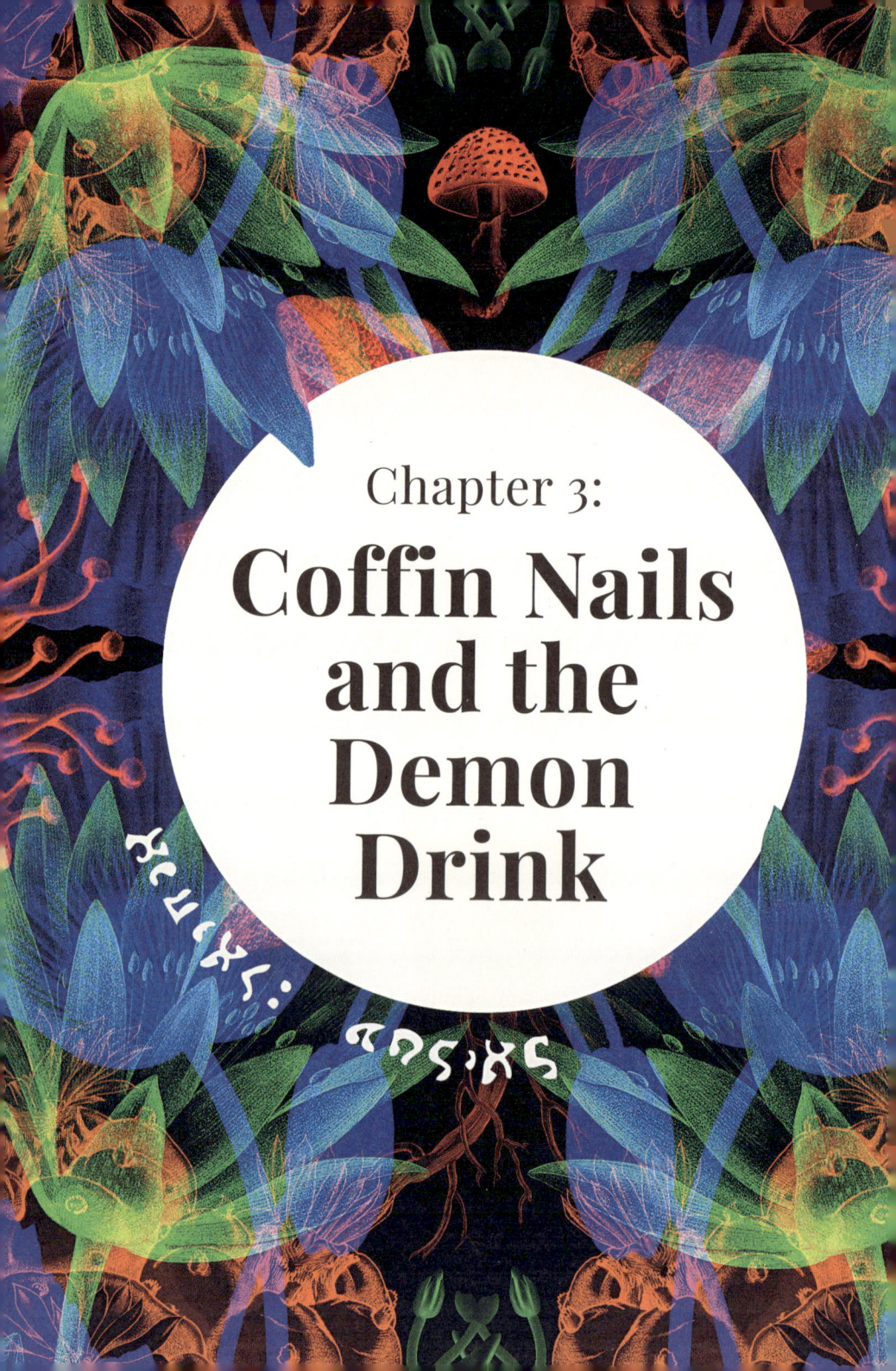

Chapter 3:
Coffin Nails and the Demon Drink

Gaspers, coffin nails, cancer sticks…
Everyone knows cigarettes are bad
news, but when you're addicted,
you're addicted, and bravado is
sometimes the best defence.
A similar gallows humour applies
to alcohol. In slang we don't get
drunk, we get hammered, we get
tanked, wasted, plastered, wrecked,
mattressed. These terms are modern
– no older than twentieth century at
most – but the folklore of smoking
and drinking, unlike almost every
other drug in this book, has always
had a darkly jovial attitude to the
perils of intoxication.

Liquid Courage: Alcohol

The Aztecs told a salutary tale of the Centzon Tōtōchtin,
400 naughty rabbit gods who spent their days
permanently plastered.

Each divine rabbit – the offspring of Mayahuel, the goddess of *pulque* (agave wine), and Petecatl, the god of medicine – represented one of the infinite ways alcohol can intoxicate, but all did not end well. After accidentally killing the god of war's mother, they were hunted down and fell victim to variously hideous deaths.

Ethanol, the ingredient in alcoholic drinks, occurs naturally during fermentation, as the sugars in organic substances are broken down by microorganisms such as yeast and bacteria. Most alcoholic drinks were once plants, rarely psychoactive in themselves, but powerful intoxicants when transformed to ethanol.

Nearly all cultures use or have used alcohol since ancient times, either in a ceremonial or spiritual capacity or as part of social interaction. The people of Mali honoured Yasigi, the dancing goddess of beer, while the ancient Greek Oenotropae enjoyed the gift of turning anything into wine. In Norse mythology, Aegir the giant brews the finest beer in the Nine Worlds, ever since his best customer, Thor, stole a massive cauldron for him. Aegir's underwater drinking hall has mermaid bartenders and drinking horns that refill themselves.

There is no sugar-coating one fact: ethanol is a killer. Absorbed through the lining of the stomach, it

reaches the brain in five minutes and starts to affect it in ten. Intoxication begins as the liver fails to keep up with the workload.

At first everything becomes slower, including reaction time and judgement. The brain releases dopamine, a chemical associated with pleasure, bringing sensations of relaxation and confidence, even as the imbiber's reasoning, memory and motor skills deteriorate. Individuals, like the Aztec rabbits, react in many different ways. They might experience blurred vision or slurred speech, mood swings, impaired judgement, nausea, confusion and/or difficulty doing simple things. They may become unruly or aggressive or remain pleasantly cheery. Continued consumption can lead to stupor, coma and even death.

All these effects have been known forever, yet in folklore, tradition and mythology, drinking is usually regarded as humorous. Hundreds of tales of tipsy gods, drunken goddesses and alcoholic folk heroes generally focus on jolly clowns and romantic villains, even into modern times. During America's Prohibition years (1920–33) gangsters supplied speakeasies, fuelling the Jazz Age. The most famous of all, Al Capone, was a ruthless murderer, but actively fashioned himself on Robin Hood. And for the down-and-outs of Depression-hit Chicago, supplied with soup kitchens and handouts by Capone courtesy of his ill-gotten gains, he may indeed have been as heroic as the legendary man in Lincoln green.

Opposite Fancy a drink? Men drinking at a speakeasy bar in 1920.

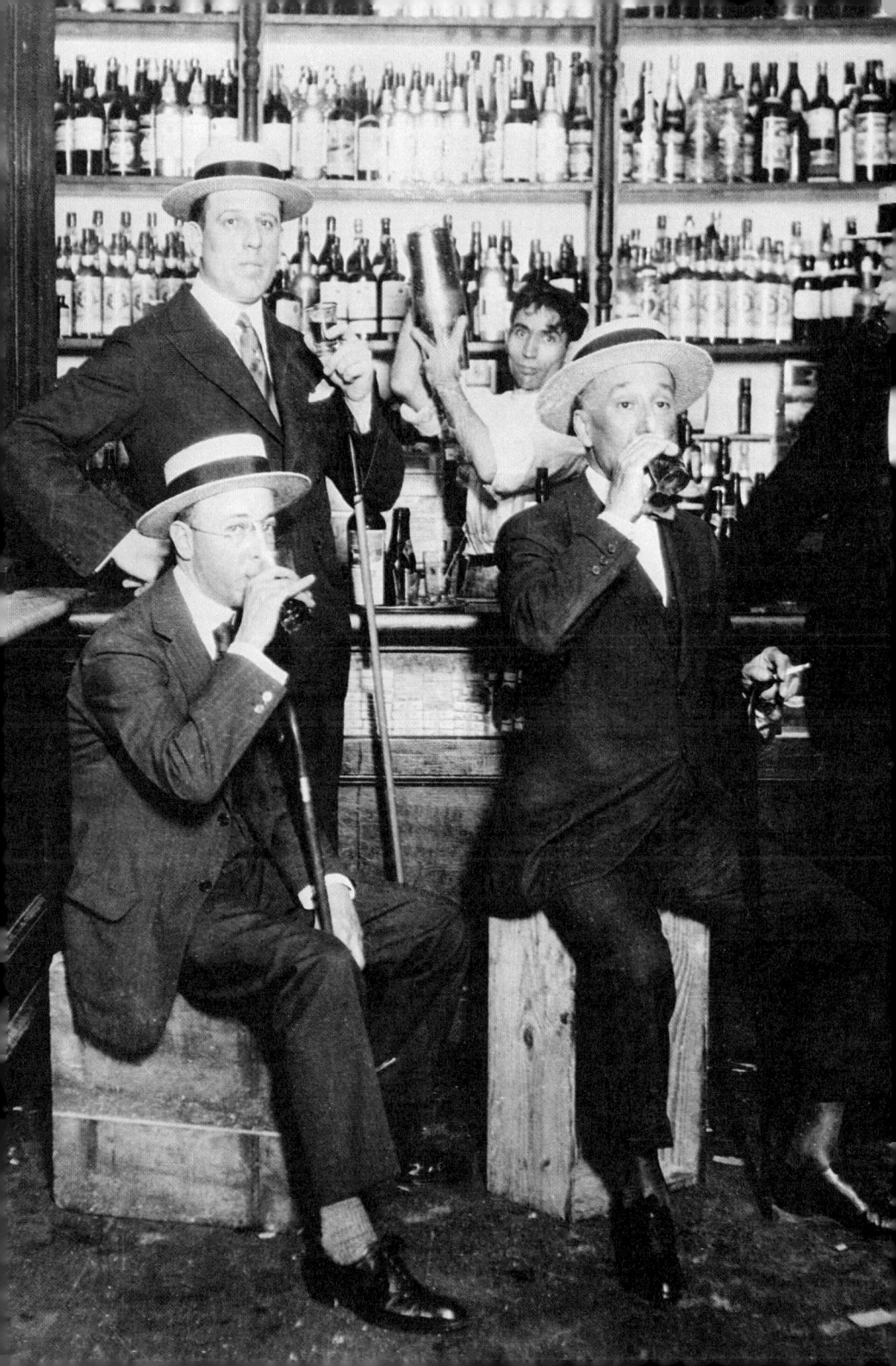

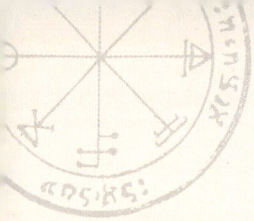

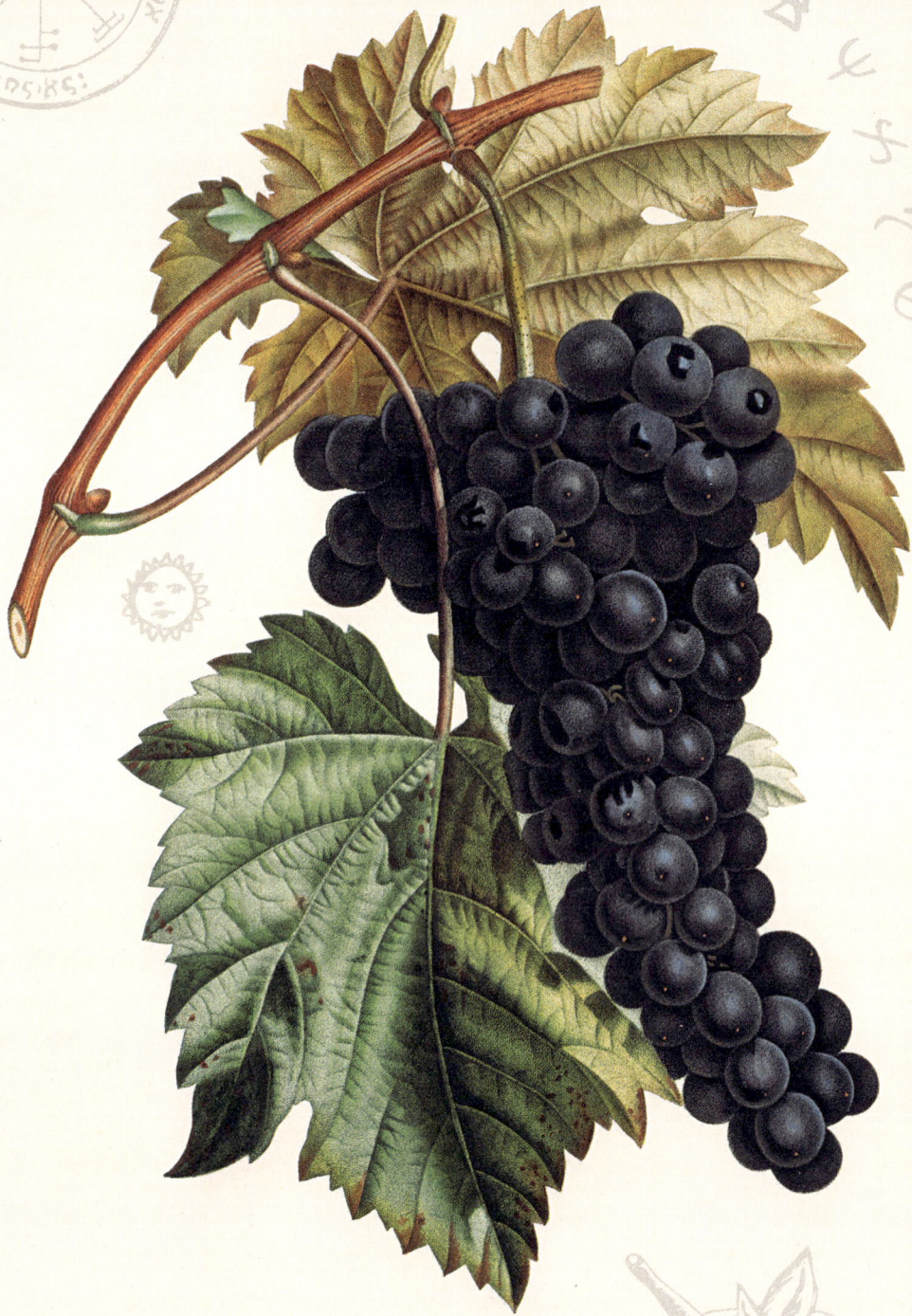

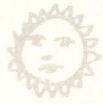

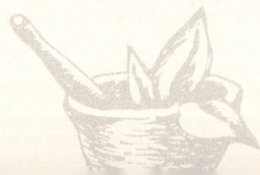

Grape

Vitis vinifera

The centrepiece of every classic cornucopia (horn of plenty) in art, as well as the plaything of satyrs and the crown of Dionysus, the grapevine has been the king of fruits since antiquity.

It is no coincidence that Dionysus and his Roman counterpart, Bacchus, are the gods of both wine and pleasure. Alcohol, especially in the form of wine, is a drug of sociability, of human connection and celebration. Yet according to Greek mythology, the vine itself was born out of grief. Dionysus's lover Ampelos tried to ride a wild bull, which tossed him from its back, instantly killing the beautiful youth. The devastated god transformed his lost love into the first grapevine.

More playfully, the ancient Greeks also loved Silenus, the permanently drunken god of winemaking, usually depicted slouched on his donkey or being held upright by equally inebriated satyrs. Balding men with cartoon-like features, the hairy legs and tails of goats, and giant erections, satyrs constantly harassed the maenads ("raving ones"), nymphs brought to a state of divine ecstatic trance though intoxication, most famously during the Mysteries of Dionysus. One of the most puzzling secrets of ancient Greece, the Mysteries are still unfathomable today, but some scholars suggest the wine served at the rites was mixed with hallucinogenic plants.

From such rich mythology, it is easy to assume that the ancient Greeks were master winemakers, but although they were fond of their thick, sweet, syrupy drink, this was not wine as we would know it. They had to water it down to render it palatable. At a symposium – always held after a banquet, upper-class and all-male (save for flute girls and courtesans) – the leader decided the dilution ratio for the evening, which usually also determined whether that night's gathering involved debate, poetry and music or became a drunken orgy.

Wine played an important role in ritual libations and, of course, the leaves and fruit were enjoyed as food. Grape vinegar – plentiful because storage was a problem and wine prone to oxidization – was used as a medicine and to flavour and preserve food.

The Romans were the first civilization to create something we would recognize as wine, learning to properly ferment the grapes, and safely store the result. By the Middle Ages vineyards were a staple of country estates and monasteries. With each harvest, techniques were further perfected.

Depending on geography and weather conditions, the all-important harvest will now commence at any time between August and November. Deciding the perfect moment requires great skill. The grapes must have their optimum balance of sugar and acid, the temperature should be cool, the atmosphere dry. The Romans had not quite worked this out when they designated specific dates for specific festivals – 19 August, *Vinalia Rustica*, petitioning Jupiter's protection for the ripening fruit in return for a slaughtered lamb; 11 October, *Meditrinalia*, the end of the harvest, when the new grape must was added to old wine to boost alcohol content; 23 April, *Vinalia Prima*, celebrating the first taste of the new wine – but these dates generally worked out well enough.

Thanks to the almost arcane nature of the harvest – every vintage is different – scores of superstitions and customs have entwined themselves around this nigh-on mystical process. Getting God on your side was important, and many cultures brought a basket of the first ripe fruit of the season into church for a blessing. Modern Greece remains typical. Some vineyards still bring a priest to lead prayers for a safe gathering on the first day of harvest, and a few continue the custom of leaving a small area uncropped as thanks for protection.

Speed is of the essence when harvesting, so almost everywhere across the wine-growing regions of Europe, the entire village – family members, friends and neighbours – turned out to help. They started very early and worked throughout the day, though stopped for a hearty lunch provided by the farmer. It was – and, in places where the harvest is still done by hand, remains – hard, joyous work, involving popular songs, laughter and ribaldry. Everyone looks forward to the traditionally huge evening meal taken together, a reward for their labour and good humour. In a few parts of Germany, the superstition of bringing in the last of the harvest in an ox-pulled cart persists, preventing the crop being filled with sour grapes.

In ancient times, crushing grapes into must (juice) with bare feet was overseen by the Treader – Silenus's demigod son Leneus, the leader of the dance of the wine trough. Tradition, however, soon assigned the task to women, and in some cultures – for example in certain regions of Portugal – it was positively unlucky for men to join in. A powerful feminine rite, the work party was often accompanied by popular "harvest songs" to ensure even treading at a specific pace.

Some places still "stomp". In Spain *pisado de la uva* festivals now invite anyone who turns up – male, female, young and old – to get inside the vat and enjoy some good, dirty fun.

Opposite An oil painting of Bacchus, the Roman god of agriculture, wine and fertility, by Caravaggio dating back to 1598.

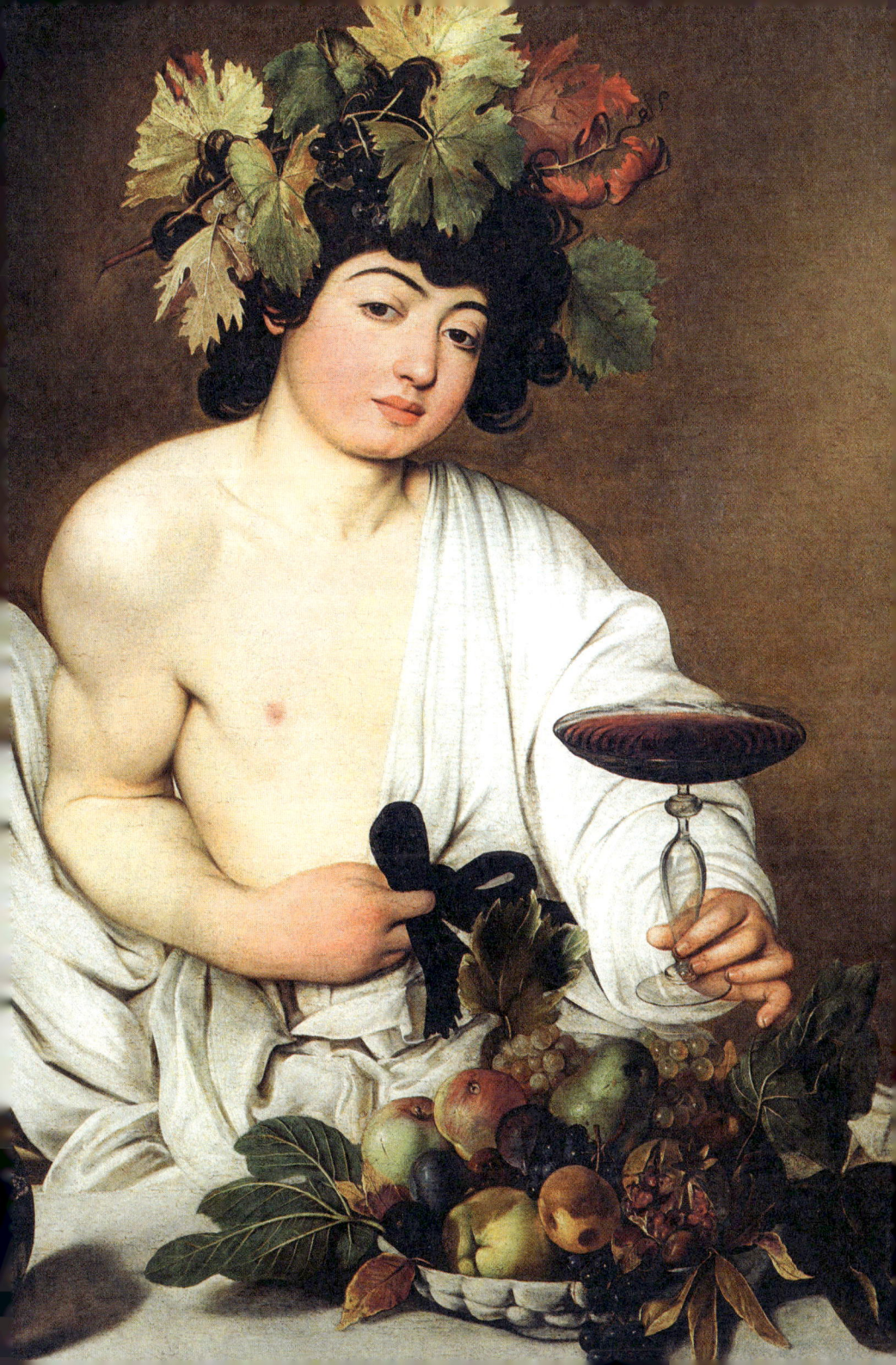

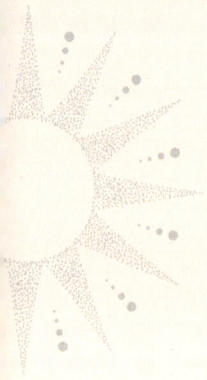

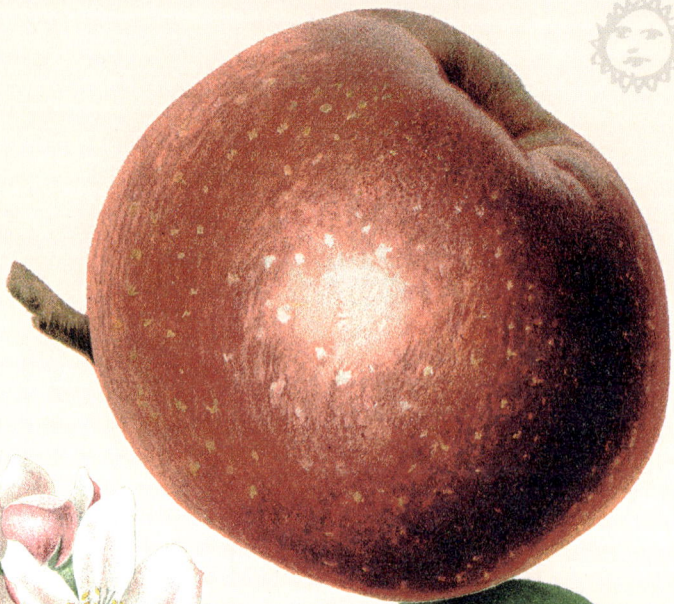

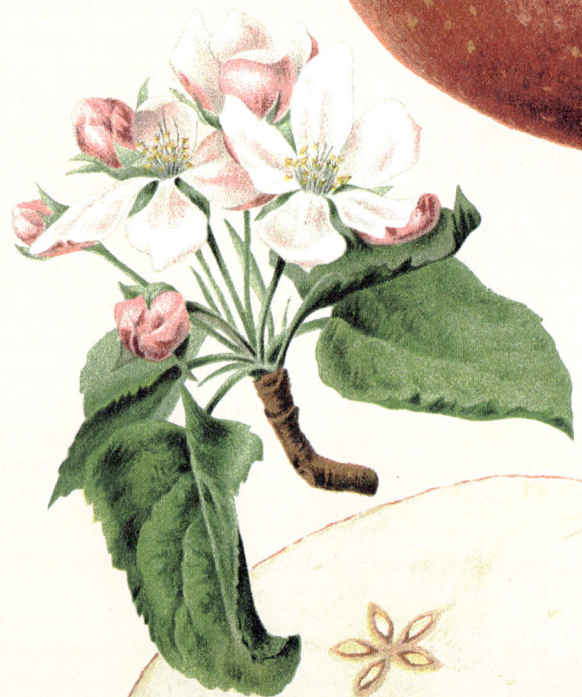

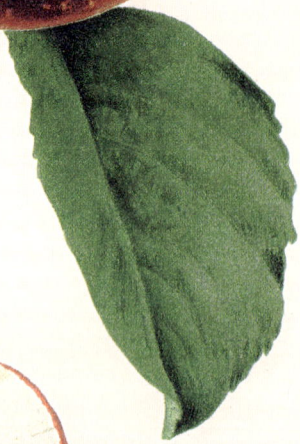

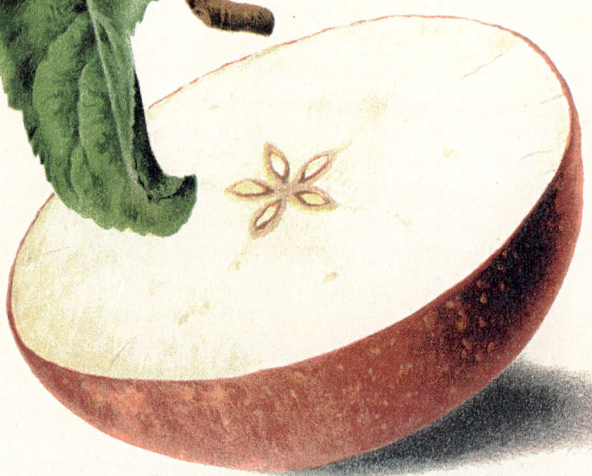

Apple

Malus

Alcohol is often blamed for people "seeing things".
One of the worst "things" a scrumper (apple thief) risks
encountering is Awd Goggie, the fearsome protector
of northern English apple orchards.

A wd Goggie is a classic "nursery bogey" who frightens children from doing silly things. His coworker, Lazy Laurence, who haunts England's more southern orchards, gives young scrumpers bellyache for eating unripe fruits. Laurence sometimes lives in the oldest tree in the orchard, sometimes he is the oldest tree, though in Somerset such a tree is just known as the Apple Tree Man. Whoever he is, Oldest Tree must be cared for, to ensure the health of the entire orchard. If properly respected, he may even reward the worthy.

Apples are among the world's earliest cultivated foods. While the remains found by ancient Egyptian archaeologists cannot definitively be linked to cider production, we know the ancient Greeks indulged. By the time the Romans invaded Britain in 43 CE, the Celts had been making an alcoholic brew from crab apples for three thousand years. Britain's Norman invaders, who arrived in 1066, enjoyed cider, too – naming it *sidre*, ultimately deriving from the Hebrew *šēkār*, or "strong drink".

By the Middle Ages, it had spread to Yorkshire, Worcestershire, Herefordshire and Somerset, still some of the great cider-producing counties. Also known as "scrumpy", the beverage kept workers going during the day, and was as popular as beer in other regions, often representing part of a labourer's wages.

As one of the most important crops, apple production attracted dozens of customs and superstitions. The sun shining through the branches on Old Christmas Day indicated a good future harvest, but just to make sure, the apple year began with wassailing (hailing) the trees, a boisterous event also known as "howling". Village lads processed through orchards discharging firearms, shouting, dancing, banging pots and pans, singing and blowing cows' horns to frighten away evil spirits, and then hit the trees with sticks and anointed them with cider. Later in the year, a more formal blessing of the trees took place on St Swithin's or St James's Day.

Alcoholic cider was hugely popular in Colonial America; the semi-legendary missionary and nurseryman Johnny Appleseed planted cider apples, not the eating variety. The drink's popularity waned with the Industrial Revolution and cheap grain prices, grinding to a near halt when hundreds of orchards were razed during Prohibition. Today, American "apple-cider" is a non-intoxicating fruit juice, though the classic alcoholic beverage is beginning to gain popularity once more.

Rice

Oryza sativa

For a society renowned for formality and tradition, Japan has a distinctly easy-going attitude to inebriation. Alcohol is not regarded as a drug and intoxication is joyfully indulged as a safety valve for a polite people living cheek by jowl.

If not celebrating *bōnenkai* ("year forgetting party"), its successor *shinnenkai* ("New Year party") or any of the five sekku (seasonal drinking parties), Japanese people will meet after work to drink with colleagues. The country does not have a traditional grape industry, so the alcohol of choice is rice wine. *Sake* is a general term for alcohol, so it is important to ask for specific wines according to the season or celebration. *O-toso* is a spiced New Year sake, and *Hanamizake* a sweet, fragrant version reserved for springtime Hanami (flower viewing), while *Tsukimizake* and *Yukimizake* are drunk at, respectively, Moon viewings and snow viewings.

Like many so many things the Japanese have made their own, rice wine originated in China. Evidence suggests *Oryza sativa* was domesticated around 9,000 years ago. *Mijiu* (Chinese rice wine) dates back to around 1000 BCE. Origin stories and dates are vague. Did a man called Jukyu really discover alcohol after smelling something strange and spotting a bamboo stump that birds had packed full of glutinous rice? Maybe it was Mijanojon, who travelled to Silla, an ancient Korean kingdom, to learn the secrets of fermentation, or Mokhwasobimae, who chewed rice in his mouth, inventing the process.

Mijiu still plays an important role in China. It is drunk warm, as is the Korean version, *cheongju*, and, of course, Japanese sake, where consumption has become a ritual. A gathering's host pours for the guest of honour; other guests serve each other. No one serves themselves, which is *tejaku*, the height of bad manners. When every *ochoko* (cup) is filled, all drink together, using both hands to hold the tiny cup.

Another Chinese import, *Kyokusui* ("winding-stream party") was celebrated on the third day of the third lunar month. Participants had to compose a traditional tanka poem in the time it took their cup of sake to float down an artificial stream. They then either drank the wine as celebration of their amazing verse or as forfeit for terrible poetry. Drinking games remain a large part of Japanese culture to this day. One of the jobs of *maiko* (apprentice geisha) is to relax guests by drinking and playing silly games.

Every Japanese celebration involves sake, whether as part of a Shinto wedding, at a *Jotoshiki* (pillar-raising ceremony) on the first day of construction, or at the opening of a new building. Many such occasions necessitate a *kagami birraki* – the ritual of breaking open a new cask of sake with a mallet, bringing good fortune to all.

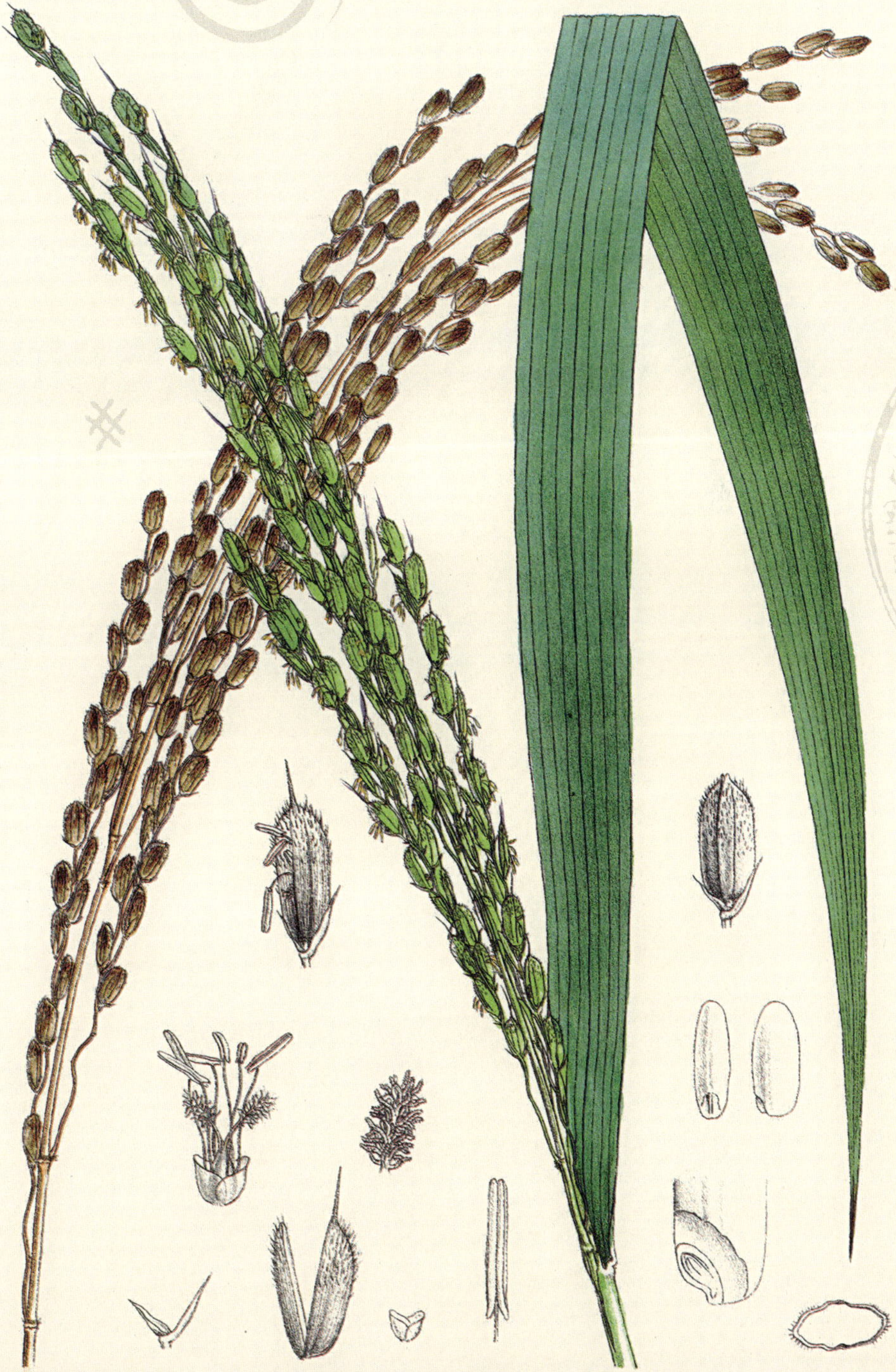

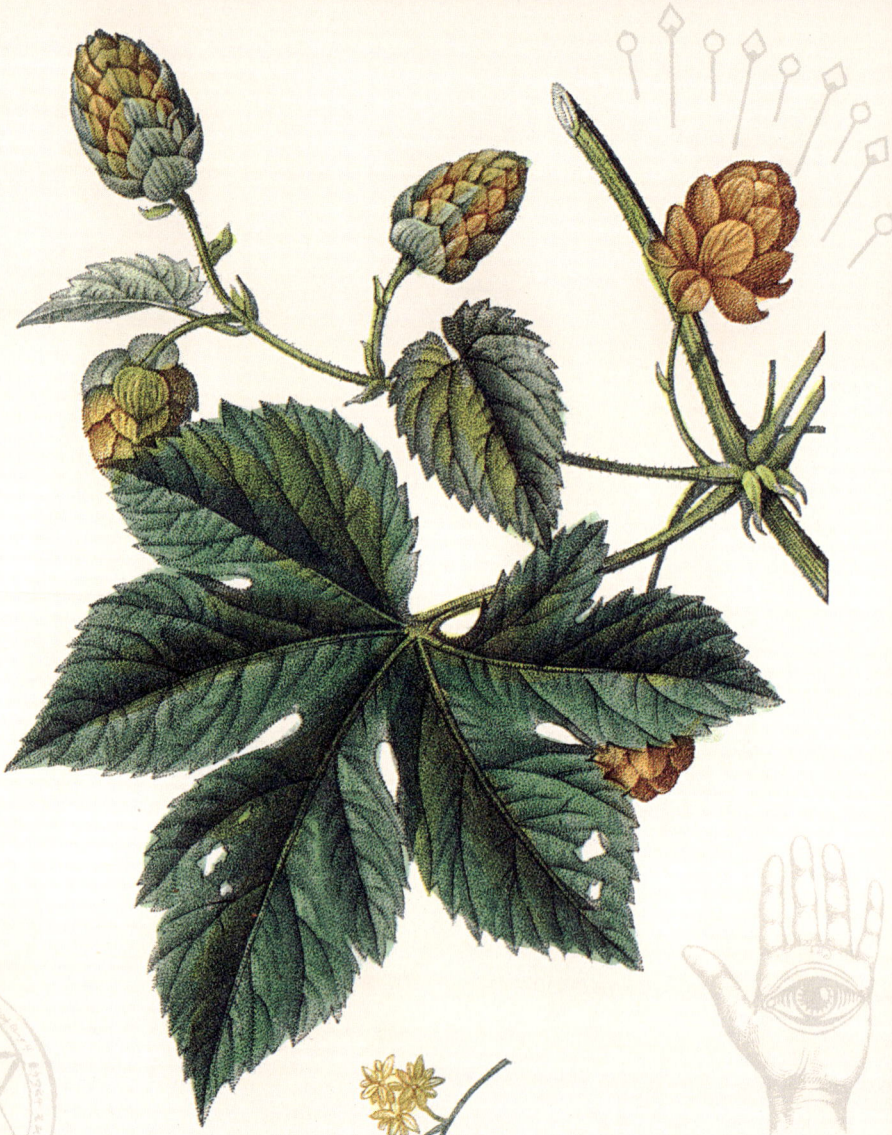

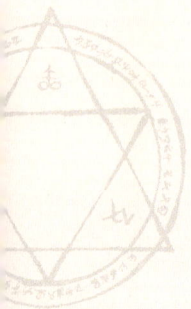

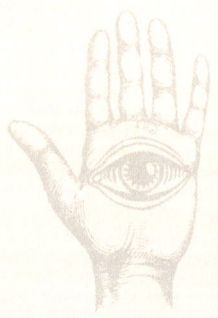

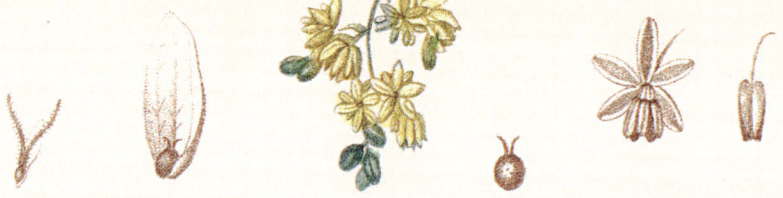

Hop

Humulus lupulus

Hearty fifteenth-century English drinkers were unconvinced when newfangled continental "beer" arrived on their shores. Happy with their Anglo-Saxon ale, they were slow to appreciate the bitter flavour lent by the hops.

Beer has been with humanity since at least ancient Egypt and Mesopotamia. The oldest-known recipe has been preserved in a poem, c. 1800 BCE, celebrating Ninkasi, the Sumerian goddess of brewing. It involved wheat berries, yeast, date syrup and barley dough – but no hops.

The idea of using hops as a flavouring first saw light in the ninth century CE, but using them as a preservative was not perfected until the thirteenth century, when German brewers finally made a beer that could last long enough to be exported. Hopped beer travelled to Flanders, the Netherlands and, finally, to England. The English traditionally drank ale – a sweeter, un-hopped malt brew – but despite early, and sometimes violent, misgivings, they eventually settled down and started brewing their own versions. By the nineteenth century "a pint of bitter" (one of several British pale ales using different balances of malt and hops) became one of the most frequent requests in in a classic British pub.

Brewers originally imported dried hops, but these were so frequently adulterated with leaves, stalks, dust, straw, sand and sundry "wood dross" that it seemed best to just grow them from scratch. The industry reached its zenith in 1867 with the opening of the magnificent, 11-storeyed Hop Exchange just south of London Bridge, then waned as pasteurization and the availability of clean water saw fewer hops required. These are now added, mainly for flavour. Hop-growing regions shrank to the West Midlands and southeastern counties, but here they took on an almost mythical status.

Hop picking required a vast army of itinerant workers, including Irish, Scottish or Romani travellers. Famously, East and Southeast London practically emptied each summer as entire families went "hopping", the closest they'd get to an annual holiday. Adults, often wearing stilts, harvested hops from tall poles connected by wires while their children ran ahead, clearing away the dead vines. Giant basketsfuls of hops were dried in oast houses, many of which still exist, mainly in Kent. Living in makeshift huts and cooking outside, hoppers worked hours that were long and hard, but their experiences have somehow taken on a rosy glow within cockney mythology.

England still enjoys a romantic relationship with the hop, as any country pub bedecked with garlands of dried hops "for luck" will attest.

Wormwood

Artemisia absinthium

Possibly the most notorious of all alcoholic drinks, absinthe has
a reputation for inducing madness – a dynamic traditionally
attributed to thujone, a neurotoxin found in wormwood,
suggested to be hallucinogenic.

Dancing a heady cancan with other romantic mythologies of Paris in the nineteenth century, the "green fairy" and her bitter taste whispered of danger and mystery, but also of creativity. Absinthe was associated with "mad genius", whether artist, author or playwright, its hallucinations facilitating new artistic highs.

Wormwood's scientific name *Artemisia* is from Artemis, Ancient Greek goddess of the Moon. The herb was known medicinally to the ancient Egyptians, mentioned in the Ebers Papyrus, though evidence of its use in alcohol has not filtered down the ages.

Wormwood leaves were soaked in wine to help with childbirth in ancient Greece, though Hippocrates also considered it useful for menstrual pain, jaundice and rheumatism, and Roman historian Pliny the Elder describes chariot-race champions drinking wormwood-infused wine.

Some suggest that absinthe was "discovered" by French troops abroad after spiking their wine with the wormwood they had been given against fever and dysentery. Back home it became fashionable to ask for *une verte* (a green) and soon drinking absinthe during *l'heure verte* (green hour) was a national pastime.

In the 1860s the phylloxera louse hit the world's vineyards, devastating the French wine industry. Cheap and quickly made, absinthe filled the somewhat dangerous gap, just as the bohemians of Paris were becoming the nineteenth-century equivalent of influencers. Degas, Van Gogh and Toulouse-Lautrec all lost themselves to the green fairy, occasionally waking up long enough to paint something.

Gradually, the drink gained a less pleasant reputation as producing a syndrome called "absinthism", involving madness, hallucinations, hyperactivity and violence. By 1880, you had only to ask the bartender for *une correspondence*, slang that was itself shorthand for *une correspondence pour Charenton* ("a ticket to Charenton"), the infamous Parisian lunatic asylum. Eventually, after a couple of high-profile drink-related murders, countries began to ban absinthe, though France didn't until the First World War, and it was never banned in Britain.

In truth, the tiny quantities of thujone typically present in absinthe are unlikely to have much toxic effect. Absinthe was often full of adulterants such as copper sulphate, antimony and aniline green, but what almost certainly caused the chaos was a combination of hysteria and good, old-fashioned alcohol poisoning.

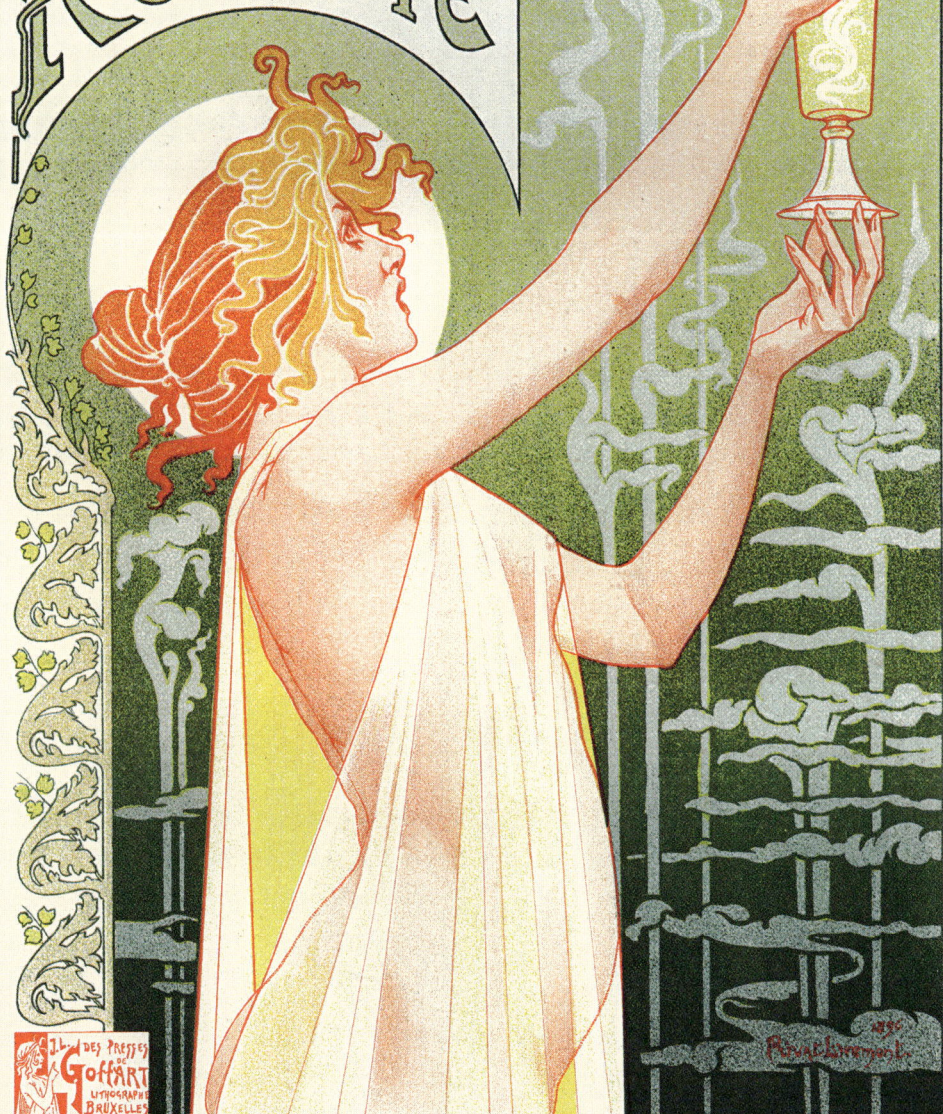

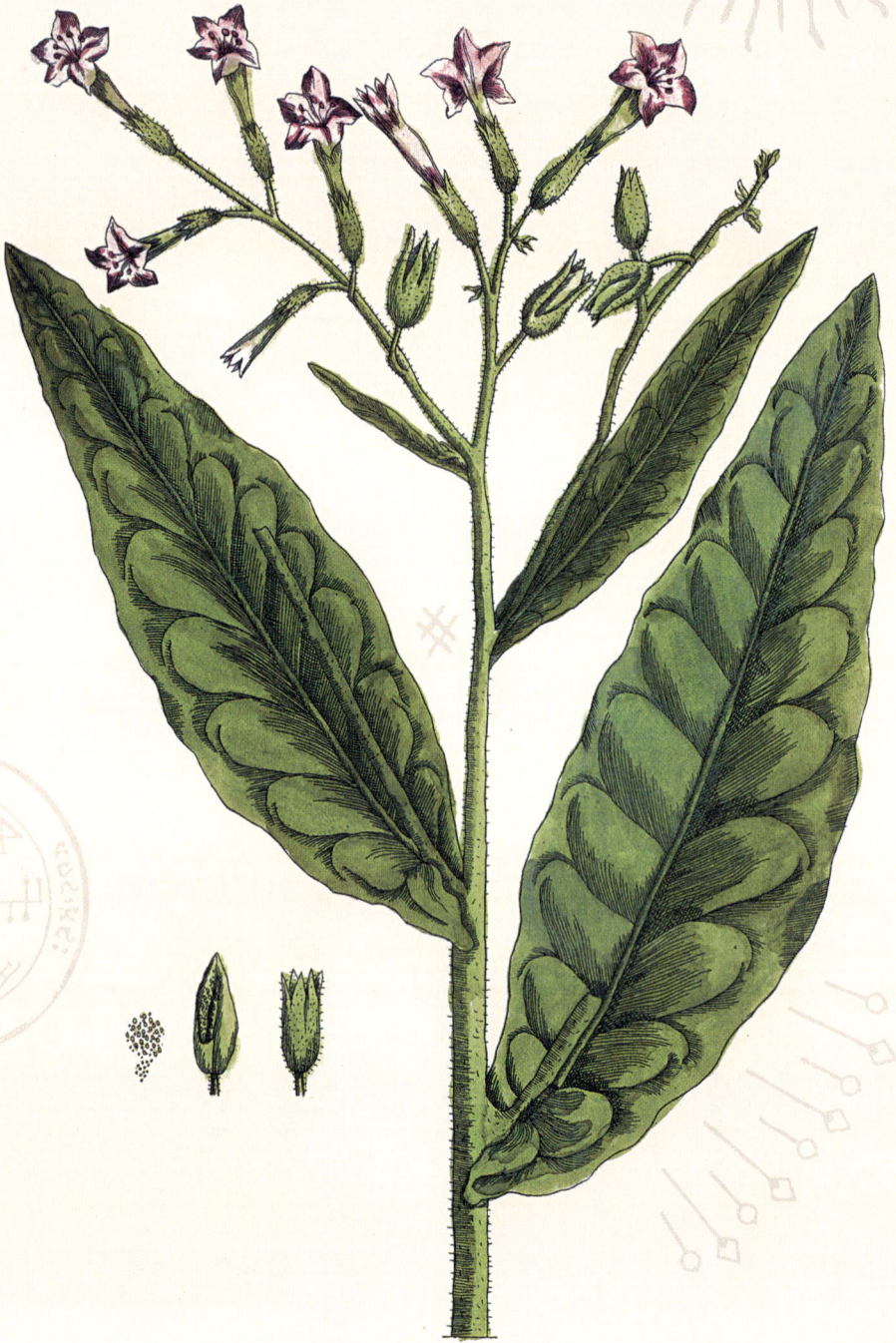

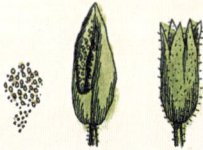

The Filthy Weed: Tobacco

A Cherokee legend tells how the white-breasted
American Dagûl'kû geese stole the only tobacco plant
in the world. Everybody suffered, but one elderly woman
was particularly poorly.

All the animals in turn tried to retrieve the plant, but each was defeated. Eventually a tiny hummingbird offered to try his luck. No one believed anyone so small could survive the quest, but Hummingbird was so fast that he had darted in and out of the Dagûl'kûs' lair before they knew what had happened. He blew smoke into the old woman's nostrils and she revived, crying out, "Tsalu!" ("Fire in the Mouth!"). Tobacco has been called Fire in the Mouth ever since.

Virtually every North American First Nation seems to have its own tobacco story, even if the plant itself appears to have derived from two wild species – *Nicotiana sylvestris* and *N. tomentosiformis*, native to Bolivia. Perhaps a peace-loving elder who promised to return after his death to remind people of brotherhood between nations really did come back as a tobacco plant, as the Nipmuck suggest, or the plant really did grow from the ashes of strange hostile beings that had raided a Haudenosaunee camp, inspiring the strongest warriors to trap and burn them. This last story is unusual, as tobacco is usually considered a plant of magic and peace. It may be used to fumigate ritually important items and spaces or shared via a peace pipe. Even the smoke itself connects the physical and spiritual and becomes an offering to the Great Spirit.

Tobacco is not like many substances in this book, for two reasons: it is not considered a hallucinogen, but it is highly addictive. It contains over 3,000 chemicals, some of which – nicotine, benzene, arsenic and formaldehyde, for example – are extremely poisonous. There is a reason why neonicotinoid insecticides are so deadly. Tobacco is even poisonous to the touch; field workers are often made literally sick with Green Tobacco Sickness (GTS). Eating the leaves has been linked with causing stomach cramps, sweating, breathing difficulties and even death.

And yet people have been obsessed with smoking tobacco for centuries. It may have been cultivated up to 8,000 years ago. Certainly, by the first century BCE, indigenous peoples in South America were using it medicinally and in religious ceremonies, usually in combination with other herbs. Commercial companies include additives too, but theirs tend to be chemically based.

Tobacco crossed the Atlantic with Christopher Columbus in 1492, who had received some as a gift. Not everyone loved the new habit of pipe-smoking. James VI and I, King of Scotland and then of England, hated it so much he wrote his own anti-smoking treatise in 1604, *A Counterblaste to Tobacco*. It's prescient stuff: James not only warns against the ills of the herb, claiming it harms the lungs, but rails against the dangers of passive smoking. He also, somewhat unfairly, blames the indigenous Americans, who used tobacco in different ways to chain-smoking Europeans. Not that James had much say in the matter. By now tobacco had been added to the list of commodities grown on New World plantations by enslaved workers, and when that proved profitable, Spanish and Portuguese merchants brought the industry to the West African coast, soon joined by Dutch colonists who set up plantations in South Africa. Everyone wanted a piece of the pipe, not least for its reputed health benefits. Rumour held (incorrectly, as we now know) it could cure migraines, coughs, even cancer. In

Below Walter Raleigh popularized tobacco in England. Here, he smokes an ostentatious pipe.

1665, London went tobacco crazy after someone suggested it repelled the plague. People still thought it was healthful, even into the mid-twentieth century, because the tobacco companies waged a (temporarily) very successful war against anyone telling them otherwise.

There is no "good" way to ingest tobacco. 'Baccy chewing, still popular today beyond the clichés of American Civil War soldiers, cowboys and Old West prospectors, risks oral cancers. Cigar smoking may be considered a luxury form of the humble cigarette, but it still causes any number of deaths every year, often from lung cancer. Pipes just shift the problems back to the mouth. Even tobacco's important shamanic relation, *Nicotiana rustica*, has a dangerously high nicotine content.

For all this, the world is not done with tobacco.

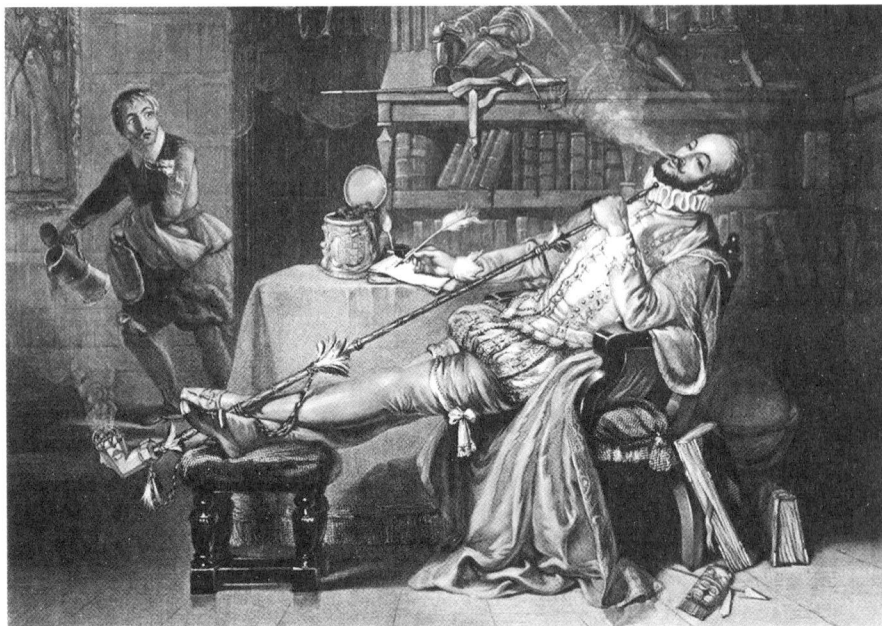

Right A 1951 US advert for Camel cigareetes, endorsed by actor and musciian Charles "Buddy" Rogers.

According to ASH (Action on Smoking and Health) legal tobacco sales are worth an estimated £605 billion each year. Deaths from smoking are estimated at around eight million per year, dwarfing every other substance in this book, including alcohol, with China's male population most at risk. We still do not know precisely what the cocktail of chemicals in commercially produced insecticides used on plants including tobacco are doing to the pollinators of the world, but more research is needed, and fast.

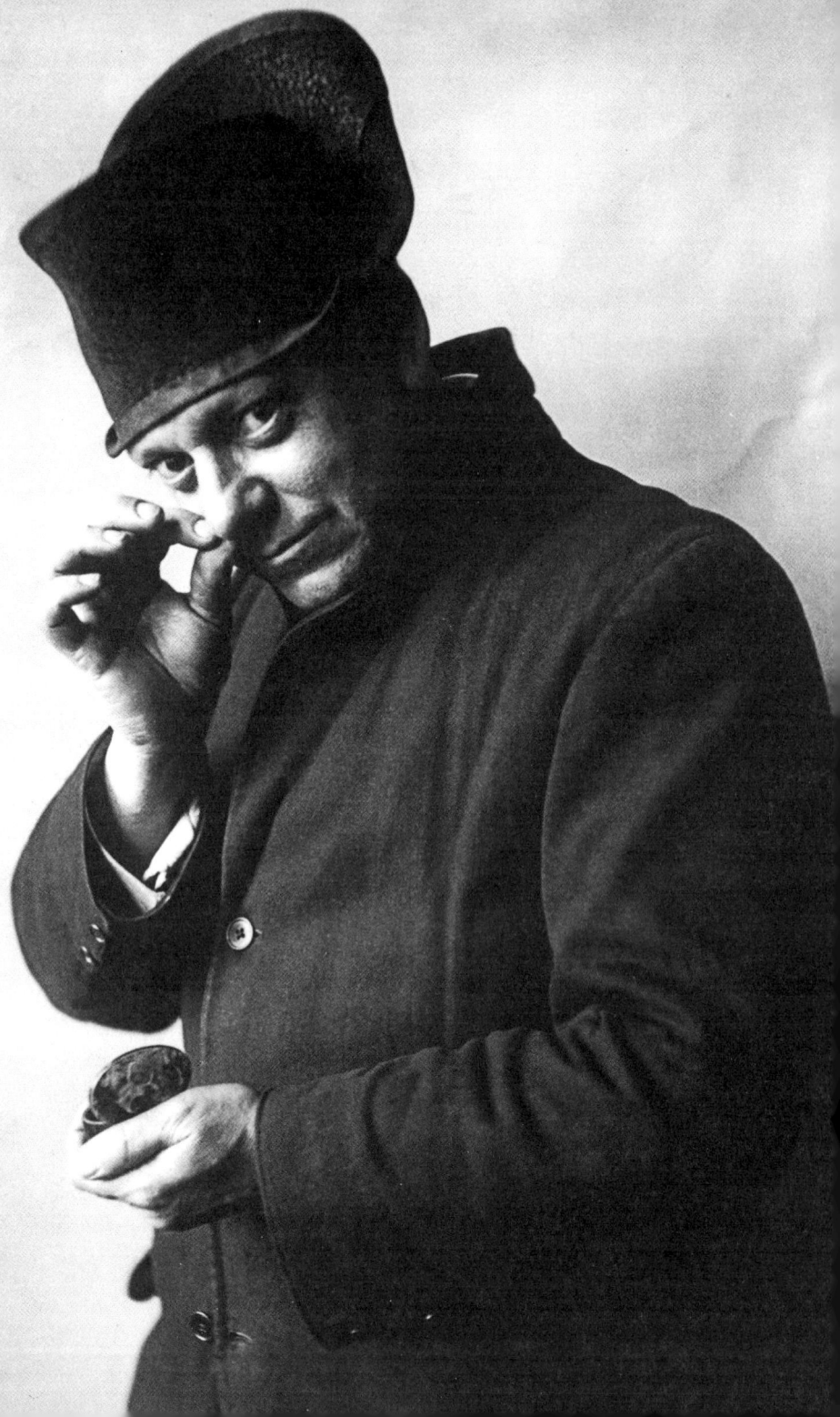

Snuff

We are in the early hours of 23 October 1702, in the heat of the Battle of Vigo Bay. English Vice Admiral Thomas Hopsonn has broken through Spanish/French lines. His enemies hastily commandeer a merchant vessel.

They set it on fire and then aim it at the *Torbay*, Hopsonn's flagship. They have, however, forgotten to check what it is carrying… a consignment of snuff, a product made from finely-ground, dried tobacco leaves, usually inhaled through the nose. The highly combustible cargo explodes, sending powder flying into the atmosphere and extinguishing the flames. The Franco-Spanish fleet was defeated, and the incident became possibly the only time snuff has actually saved lives. Then again, snuff captured from the rest of the treasure fleet was taken back home, where sniffing became a patriotic craze, so maybe not.

Not that the habit hasn't claimed to have medicinal properties. The French diplomat Jean Nicot, who has the dubious honour of being the inspiration for the word *nicotine*, introduced snuff to the French court. He taught his queen Catherine de' Medici how to finely grind the dried tobacco leaves before sniffing the result as a headache preventative. It started a fashion that spread quickly across Europe, gaining the name *snuff* from the Dutch term *snuftabak*, a contraction of the words for *sniff* and *tobacco*. By the eighteenth century *snuff* had its own panoply of regalia and etiquette – though, oddly, the South and Central American indigenous practice of

sniffing together, ceremonially blowing snuff up each other's nostrils, never really took off.

Other imported practices were warmly embraced. Just as indigenous people kept their supply in elaborate containers, snuffboxes became highly collectible. Craftsmen vied to create the most beautiful works of tiny art using gold, silver, enamelling, jewels and miniature paintings. These sometimes came with fancy ivory graters so users could grind their own. A very coarse blend called *rappee* (from the French "to grate") is still available.

Indigenous peoples mixed roots, ash, dung, herbs and other materials with the tobacco to act as a bridge between themselves and the spirits. Georgian dandies perfumed their snuff with lavender, clove, jasmine and attar of roses, in an eighteenth-century version of today's candy vapes. Women enjoyed it, too. George III's queen was so fond of a sniff she was nicknamed "Snuffy Charlotte". Carved wooden "Scottish Highlanders" stood outside snuff shops a little like American "cigar-store Indians". Read into that what you will.

The fashion didn't last – not necessarily because snuff can be as carcinogenic as any other form of tobacco, merely that more effective stimulants came along. The product still exists in Europe but is generally regarded with the same quaintness as frock coats, periwigs and quizzing glasses.

Opposite A man is pictured taking snuff circa 1900.

Thank You for Smoking – Tobacco in the Movies

Smoking has been a heavily coded image from the very earliest days of cinema. Quite apart from reflecting real life – the habit was almost universal – a cigarette managed to represent glamour, rebellion and that untranslatable something: cool.

Tobacco had another useful quality, especially when it came to the dark shadows of film noir in the 1940s and '50s. Smoke catches beautifully in carbon arc lighting, casting a mysterious veil over hero, femme fatale and master criminal alike. In *Out of the Past* (1947), Robert Mitchum's days go by "like a pack of cigarettes you smoked". Humphrey Bogart was rarely seen without his trademark smoke, and the only reason a sleepless Glenn Ford knew Rita Hayworth was brooding silently across a darkened veranda in *Affair in Trinidad* (1952) was the pulsing glow of her cigarette and a pair of haunting eyes.

The tobacco industry had been sponsoring major stars to endorse various brands in fan magazines since 1927. Most Golden Age actors smoked anyway; after all, the camera notoriously added ten pounds, and they needed something to suppress those appetites. When, a few years later, the Hays Code clamped down on – among many other things – sex, violence and drugs, tobacco became a substitute for all three. Cigarettes were most common, smoked by housewives, ingénues, gumshoes, barflies and villains alike, and occasionally appearing in sleek holders – step forward Audrey Hepburn in *Breakfast at Tiffany's* (1961). Pipes were puffed by older, trustworthy characters, while children's cartoons mainly featured cigars because they looked funnier.

As the century progressed, evidence piled up for the dangers of tobacco. Smoking became a symbol of rebellion. James Dean, on his motorcycle, cigarette hanging from his mouth; Clint Eastwood chewing a cheroot in the *Dollars Trilogy* (1964–66); even bad girl Olivia Newton-John at the end of *Grease* (1978). As smoking in public was slowly banned, cinema became more squeamish, upping the age rating on movies featuring tobacco use. "Dangerous" people still smoked – think Robert de Niro in *Goodfellas* (1990), Sharon Stone in *Basic Instinct* (1992) and Brad Pitt in *Fight Club* (1999) – but smoking by "regular" characters declined.

There was one way for the industry to have its nicotine-laced cake and eat it: period drama. In the TV series *Mad Men* (2007–15), smoking sneaked under the radar using the guise of historical authenticity, simultaneously managing to look cool, sexy and edgy while, at the same time, implying its characters would eventually suffer. The wheeze is everywhere, from biopics *Oppenheimer* (2023) and *Maestro* (2023), both depicting chain-smoking figures from recent history, to streamed series including *Stranger Things* (2016 and ongoing) and *Orange Is the New Black* (2013–19). Knowing the dangers of smoking does not seem to have lessened its appeal in Tinsel Town.

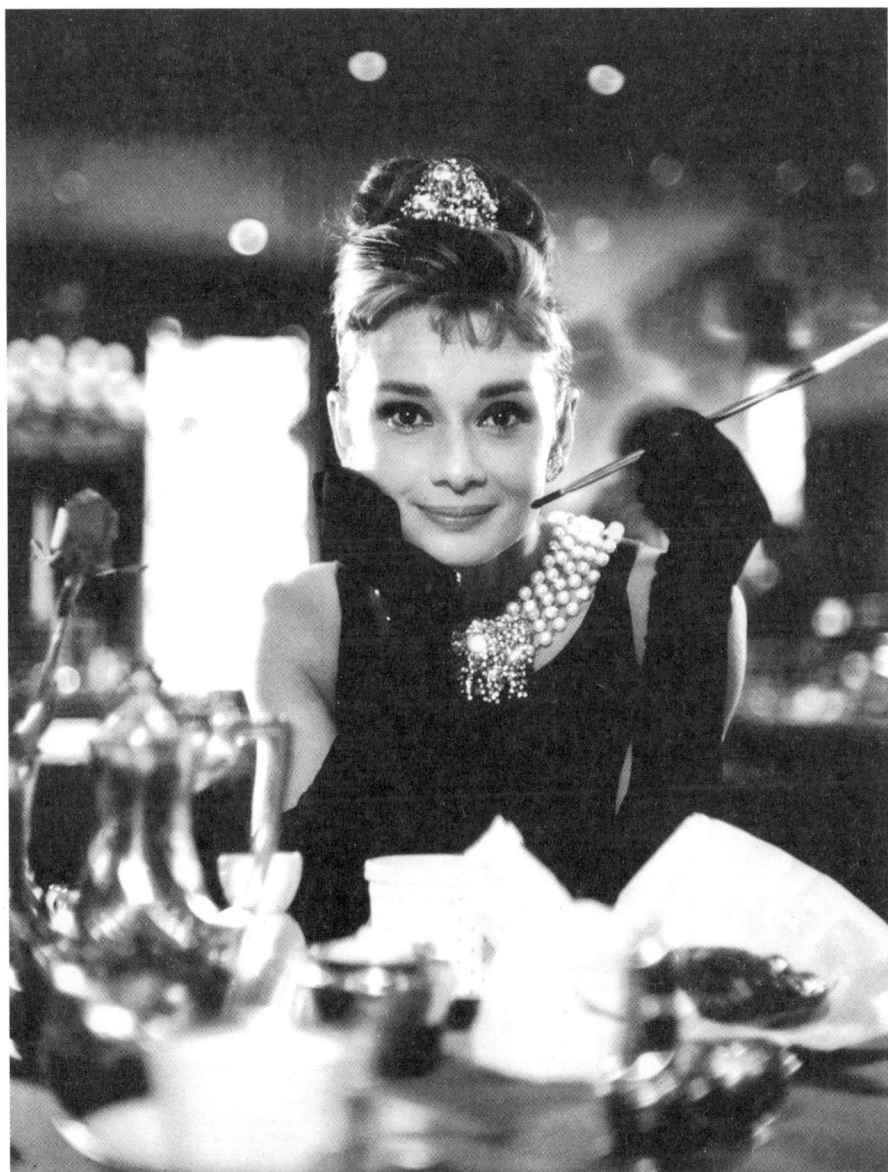

Above Audrey Hepburn smokes a cigarette using a cigarette holder in
her role as the charming Holly Golightly in *Breakfast at Tiffany's* (1961).

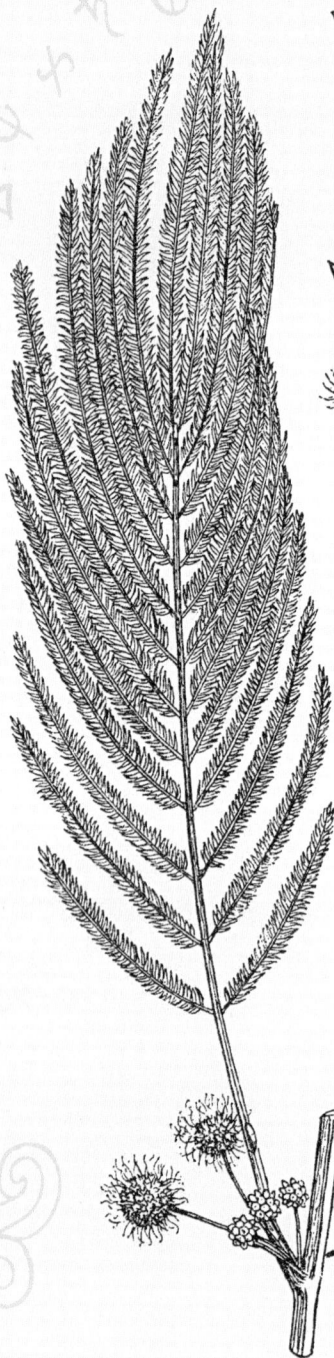

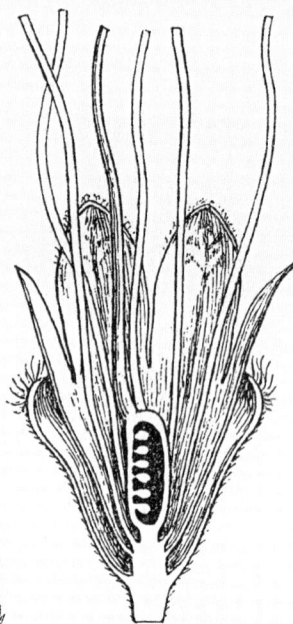

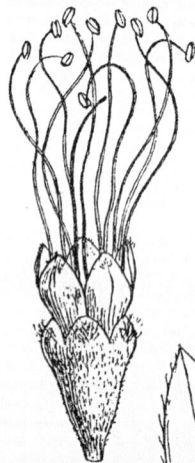

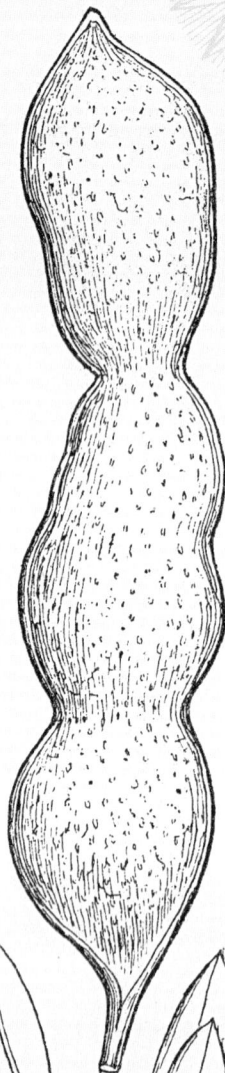

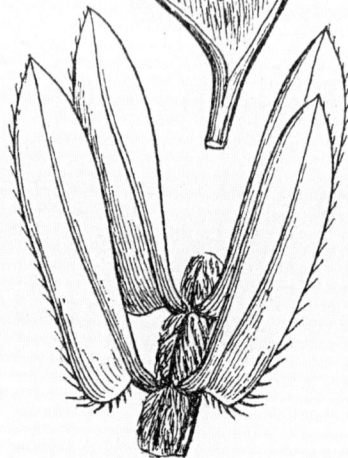

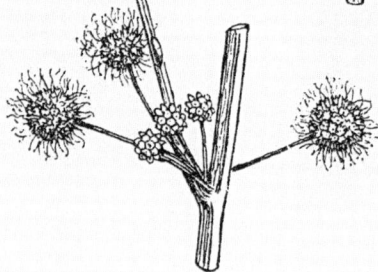

Yopo

Anadenanthera peregrina

In 1496, Ramón Pané, a friar on Columbus's second voyage to the Americas, reported an intoxicating, snuff-like herb that the Taino people of the Caribbean took into their nostrils through a long cane, resulting in hallucinations and wild behaviour.

Later missionaries were convinced users were possessed by the demons, but there was always some confusion as to which herb the various reports were referencing. Only in 1916 was the substance identified as *Anadenanthera peregrina*, used across South America under many names, including yopo.

Anadenanthera peregrina, native to northern South America, is in the pea family, producing 30cm/12in-long pods that look like strings of beads hanging between feathery, deeply pinnate leaves. Roasted and ground, the seeds make a strongly hallucinogenic snuff enjoyed across Colombia, Peru, Brazil, Venezuela and Argentina. Each community traditionally used it in their own way – to convene with the spirits, to discover the cause of an illness, to inspire courage in battle or before setting out on a hunt. Paraphernalia, including golden trays, turns up regularly on archaeological digs. Organic remains inside ceramic pipes found in northwestern Argentina, have been dated to c. 2130 BCE.

Yopo is likely to have originated somewhere around the Orinoco basin of Colombia and Venezuela, where the tree grows wild. Legend says that the Sun created the herb so humans could contact the god.

He kept the powder in his navel, where his daughter found it and gave it to people. The story has lost its context but may originate with Sué, the sun god of the Muisca community, living in the Colombian Andes before the Spanish conquest.

Yopo is generally blown through a long tube, perhaps a hollow plant stem or long-legged bird bones; chewed, allowing the compounds to be absorbed in the mouth; or smoked, for a shorter, more intense experience. Occasionally the seeds are eaten, which can result in violent ritual vomiting. The visions last around 20 minutes and tend towards flowing, often monochrome shapes. Users may also experience burning sensations, crazed delirium, unintelligible babbling and convulsive sneezing, eventually ebbing away to a trance-like stupor. It can also trigger seizures.

Anadenanthera peregrina contains a cocktail of compounds, and like everything else related to the plant, few are well understood. Its main psychoactive alkaloid is bufotenine, not dissimilar to psilocybin or the body's own compound, serotonin. Bufotenine also appears in the venom of the Bufo toad, whose venom is also psychedelic. As the best reports say, "more research is needed".

Chapter 4:
Pretty Little Poppy

In 1900 L. Frank Baum's *The Wonderful Wizard of Oz* saw young heroine Dorothy and her little dog Toto succumb to unnatural slumber in a field of magical poppies. Baum was using artistic licence – you cannot get high merely sniffing poppy flowers – but perhaps it is no coincidence that just two years earlier a different kind of heroin had hit the market, one that also sent people to sleep.

Opium poppy

Papaver somniferum

The opium poppy (*Papaver somniferum*) contains opiates: chemical compounds with narcotic properties. It packs enough punch to have remained the world's principal source of painkillers for the past few millennia.

Archaeologists have found traces of *Papaver somniferum* at Neolithic sites including central Italy, northeastern Spain and even Belgium, far from the plant's natural habitat, suggesting our ancestors knew all about its qualities. The Sumerians of Mesopotamia (western Asia) called it *Hul Gil* ("plant of joy") and passed it on to the Assyrians. In turn, they gave it to the Egyptians, who traded with the ancient Greeks. It's never looked back.

The opium poppy's distinctive seed head is a popular symbol in Greek mythology, but its meaning depends on who exactly is holding it. If Apollo or Aesculapius carry a stem or two, we are fine; they are both gods of medicine, exploiting the plant's therapeutic powers. When Aphrodite, goddess of love, sports a poppy in her crown, we are reminded of its pleasurable, supposedly aphrodisiac qualities. If Nyx, goddess of night, or her sons Hypnos (god of sleep) or Morpheus (god of dreams) hold the seed heads, expect some poppy-induced fantasy fireworks. When another of Nyx's sons gets involved, though, it is time to leave, for Thanatos is the personification of death.

The poppy's fatal properties have been known since antiquity, yet opium has also carried connotations of mercy. When the goddess Demeter lost her daughter Persephone to Hades, king of the underworld, the gods gave the distraught mother poppy to help her sleep. The Romans called her Ceres and offered her field poppies (*Papaver rhoeas*) to inspire bountiful harvests, because *Papaver somniferum* was strictly for Somnus, god of sleep. Yet all the time, the plant was also medicine, described by Dioscorides in his *De materia medica*, the most important medicinal text across many centuries.

The opium poppy's active ingredients are harvested by scoring the skin of unripe seed heads, and tapping the bitter, milky substance that flows from the wound. This turns to a brown resin, which is opium. This can be processed to isolate its opiates (the term *opioids* also includes synthetic forms). The strongest is morphine, first isolated in the early nineteenth century by German chemist F. W. Sertürner, and named for Morpheus. Along with codeine, morphine acts as an analgesic and narcotic. Papaverine, also present, has smooth muscle relaxant qualities. Opium's various alkaloids slow the body's respiration and heartbeat, and suppress

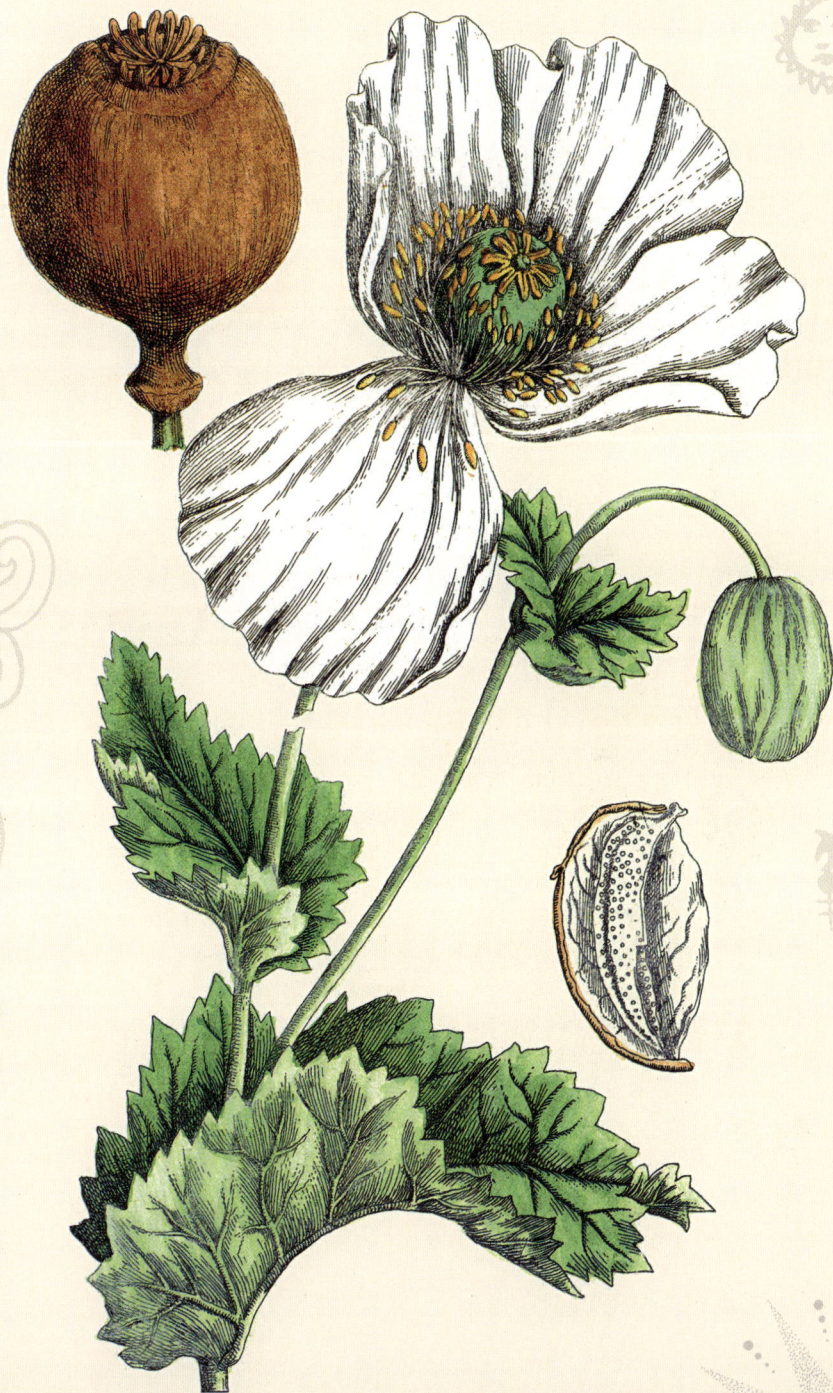

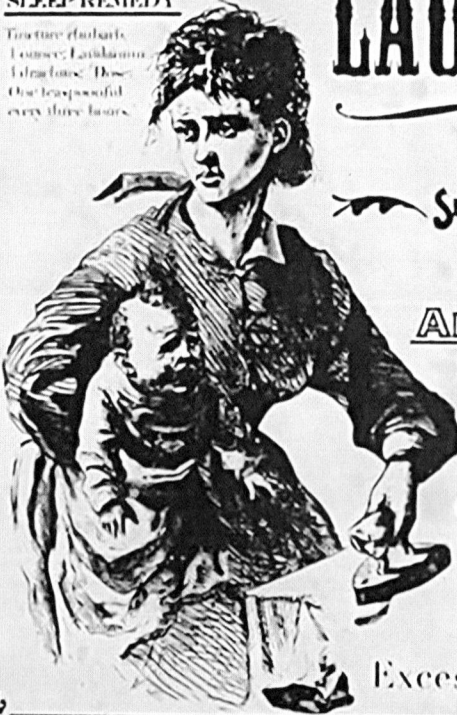

the cough reflex, making them ideal – in nineteenth-century eyes, at least – for use in cough syrups, even for children and infants.

Laudanum, an alcoholic tincture containing at least 10% opium, was an extremely popular analgesic and sedative. Dating back to the sixteenth century, the preparation was used to alleviate anxiety, suppress pain and enhance mood as a euphoric, rather than hallucinogenic drug. Its rather more unpleasant side effects – including dependency and, occasionally, death – were accepted almost as occupational hazards. They were hardly news; even John Gerard in his 1597 *Herbal*, noted: "Opium somewhat too plentifully taken doth also bring death, as Pliny truely writeth."

Medicine in the sixteenth and seventeenth centuries was a strange beast, often keeping one foot in the old astrological ways even as science progressed. The poppy was held to be variously ruled by Saturn or the Moon, and dried poppy heads were a popular folk divination medium: slip a question written on a piece of paper into the pod, pop it under your pillow, recite a charm and the answer will appear in your dreams. It was whispered that witches in Tuscany read the shapes and sizes of flames produced when they placed poppy leaves onto hot coals; other methods included consulting burnt seeds and petals. In his book *Three Books of Occult Philosophy* (1533), the sixteenth-century polymath Heinrich Agrippa includes some frankly gruesome spells for hiding gold, consulting the planets and to "make spirits and strange shapes appear". The various forms of poppy he uses seem positively tame alongside some ingredients – bats' blood, frogs' heads, cats' brains, bulls' eyes and menstrual blood – but warding off the conjured spirits was easy enough: just add "smallage" (celery) to the pot. According to folklore, throwing poppy seeds at demons would also force the bugaboos to stop and count them, enabling a swift getaway.

There was no getting away from the real-life horrors of opium, though, and these became only more intense in 1898, when a new substance, diamorphine – morphine modified with acetic anhydride – hit the pharmaceutical market. The most potent painkiller yet, "heroin" (originally a trade name) was welcomed as the latest wonder drug, but quickly lost its shine as the therapeutic benefits became outweighed by its highly addictive nature. As the twentieth century wore on, heroin was increasingly used recreationally. Tolerance levels develop quickly in users, necessitating ever-increased doses to find the same effect. What may begin as a single smoke often turns to intravenous use, carrying not only the dangers of the drug itself but complications resulting from sharing needles.

Heroin is no longer acceptable to the medical profession, but we are not yet done with opium. Morphine is still one of the strongest painkillers known to humanity, still used to bring comfort to those most severely in pain. Demeter would understand.

Opposite An advert for Laudanum, a mixture of opium and high-proof alcohol used to cure and ease a range of symptoms, in a British newspaper from around 1880.

Confessions of the Opium Eaters –
The Poppy in the Nineteenth Century

Ten thousand scimitars flash in the sunlight, and thrice ten
thousand dancing-girls strew flowers. Then follow white
elephants caparisoned in countless gorgeous colours, and
infinite in number and attendants. Still the Cathedral Tower
rises in the background, where it cannot be...

Charles Dickens's *The Mystery of Edwin Drood* begins with wicked Uncle John Jasper – choirmaster by day, poppy fiend by night – hallucinating a sultan's procession in Princess Puffer's opium den. We never find out exactly what happens, as Dickens's last novel was never finished, but that trippy opening does not bode well for Uncle Jasper's mental condition when contemplating his nephew Edwin.

By 1870, when *Edwin Drood* was published, the opium den cliché was well worn, and already on its way down the social scale. A habit once indulged by upper and lower classes alike in romantic novels now scuffed along the gutter with criminals and ne'er-do-wells in the seamier parts of town in crime stories and bodice-rippers.

For the opium poppy, the nineteenth century was the best of times, and the worst of times. On the one hand it was *the* go-to medicine, used by writers such as Walter Scott, Elizabeth Barrett Browning and Lord Byron; on the other, it fuelled two wars and an unknown number of deaths.

There was one point in its favour: opium worked. It really did soothe pain, really did relax the mind and certainly seemed to cure anything from gout to whooping cough. The Victorian pharmaceutical industry was entirely unregulated. Anyone could buy anything from any druggist – or even grocer – for pennies, and this was the age of the patent medicine. Opium was the "woman's friend", taken for everything from menstrual cramps to hysteria, sometimes, even, mixed with belladonna as "twilight sleep", allowing for childbirth with no memory of the experience afterwards. It was the "mother's friend", administered to children as Ayer's Cherry Pectoral (opium, alcohol and, perhaps, cherry flavouring to mask the taste) or Godfrey's Cordial – a subtle mix of opium, water and treacle, which certainly did keep even teething infants quiet. One Night Cough Syrup contained alcohol, cannabis, chloroform and morphine "skilfully combined with a number of other ingredients" – unnamed, presumably, because one of them might be dangerous.

Unfortunately, opium had other effects, and though the word *addiction* was not used until the twentieth century, thousands became dependent on laudanum, opium or morphine. Attitudes to this reflected class – an aristocrat formed a "habit"; for

Opposite An illustration of a woman injecting morphine from 1930. The drug was known as the "woman's friend" as it was taken to help msntrual cramps, childbirth pains and hysteria.

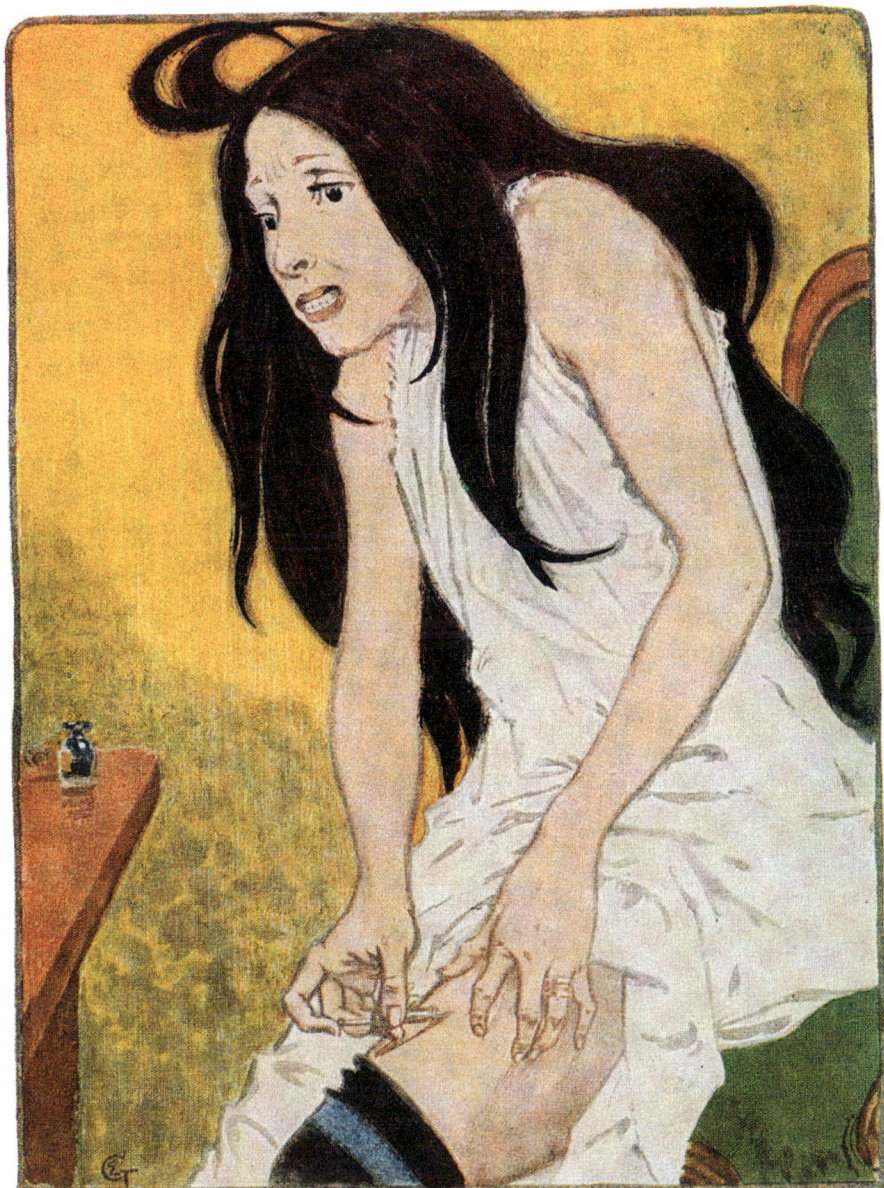

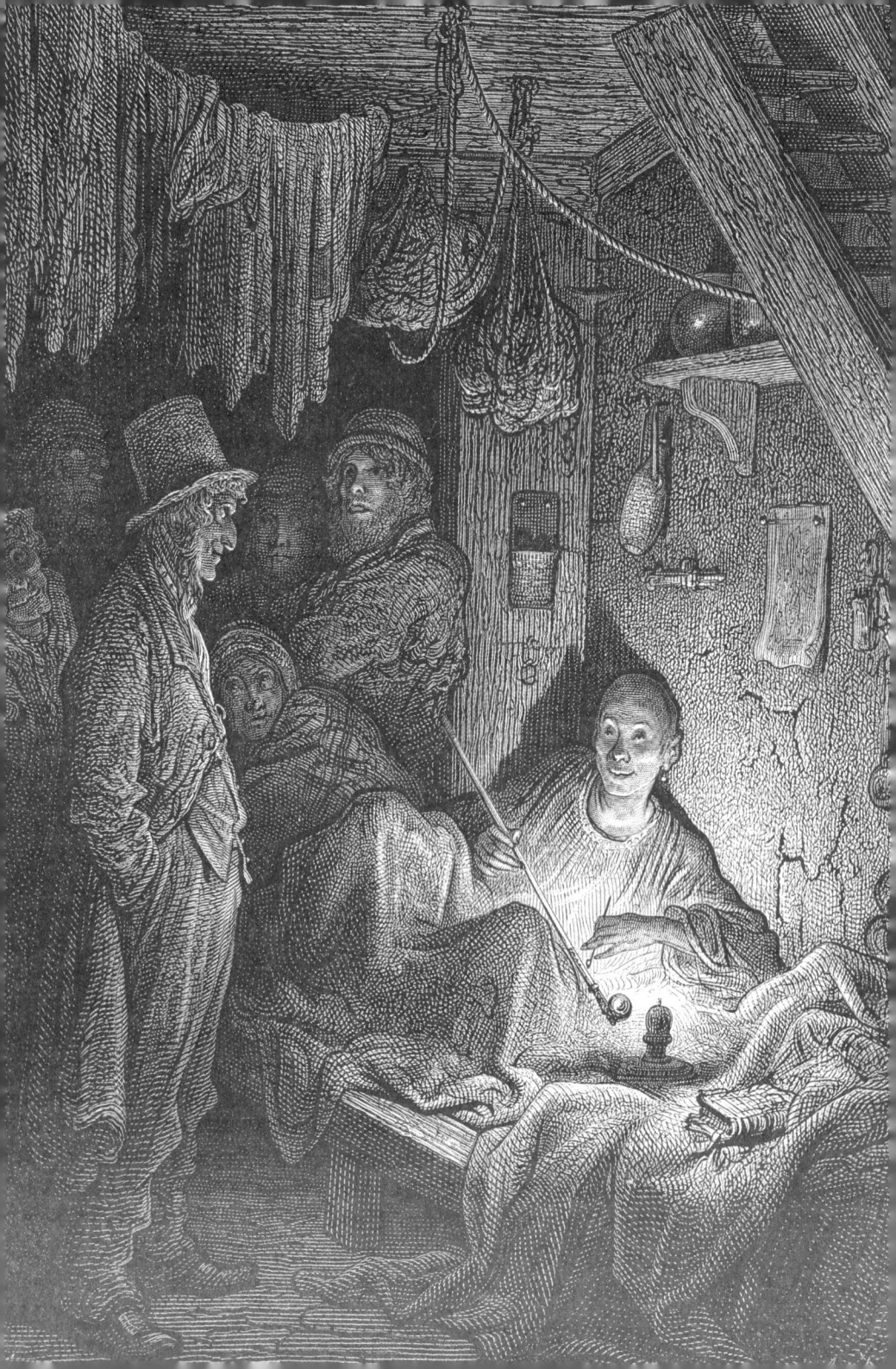

the working-class, the drug revealed an underlying character defect. Addicts experienced euphoric highs and claimed wild visions (despite opium being classed as a depressant rather than a hallucinogen), followed by profound bleakness, nausea, vomiting and craving for the next hit. Nineteenth-century literati could not get enough of it.

Elizabeth Gaskell, George Eliot and Percy Bysshe Shelley, among countless others, all used opium. Samuel Taylor Coleridge's *Kubla Khan* was based on a particularly vivid opium dream, but it was Thomas de Quincey who first wrote an autobiographical account of life as an addict, spawning a whole new genre. *Confessions of an English Opium-Eater*, published in 1821 when de Quincey was 36, is a strange book, both florid and honest, but within its frankly purple prose lies an addict's genuine desire to explain exquisite pleasure, devastating emptiness and self-revulsion to a world that does not understand. Like so many before and after, de Quincey originally took laudanum to treat excruciating rheumatic cramps, and we must remember that this was an age without other effective painkillers. The drug is, for him, both "an abyss of divine enjoyment" and "an accursed chain". He would have many literary successors – William S. Burroughs, Aldous Huxley, Hunter S. Thompson – but few capture such euphoria and despair in their work.

The opium was flowing free and fast across the British Empire, too much for the home market. Besides, people wanted pretty things, like silks and porcelain and tea – all treasures produced by the Chinese. Unfortunately, the West had nothing the Chinese wanted in return, so the British (and other imperial powers) began smuggling opium to China illegally. By 1842 the resulting addiction epidemic was becoming a national emergency. The Chinese government determined to do something about it, openly taking on the might of the British Empire who, alongside France, fought two mighty Opium Wars (1839–42; 1856–60). The Chinese were routed, lost much land (including Hong Kong) and were forced to legalize opium, which remained a serious problem.

Back home, people were finally beginning to realize that opium was not quite the wonder drug they had been peddled. A new painkiller, aspirin, had appeared, with fewer unpleasant side effects, and in 1888 Benjamin Broomhall founded the snappily titled Christian Union for the Severance of the Connection of the British Empire with the Opium Traffic, harnessing a growing anti-opium movement.

The vices presented by opium dens became ever more thickly sensationalized – often, without the slightest whiff of irony, depicted as the vice of "Orientals". This racist stereotype would reach its distasteful zenith with Sax Rohmer's opium-den-dwelling supervillain Dr Fu Manchu terrorizing London's Docklands. The first novel was published in 1913, just in time for the First World War when, in yet another irony, opium would be needed more than ever.

Opposite Opium is a depressant, causing drowsiness when smoked, so opium dens became popular places to stock the drug and tools to use it.

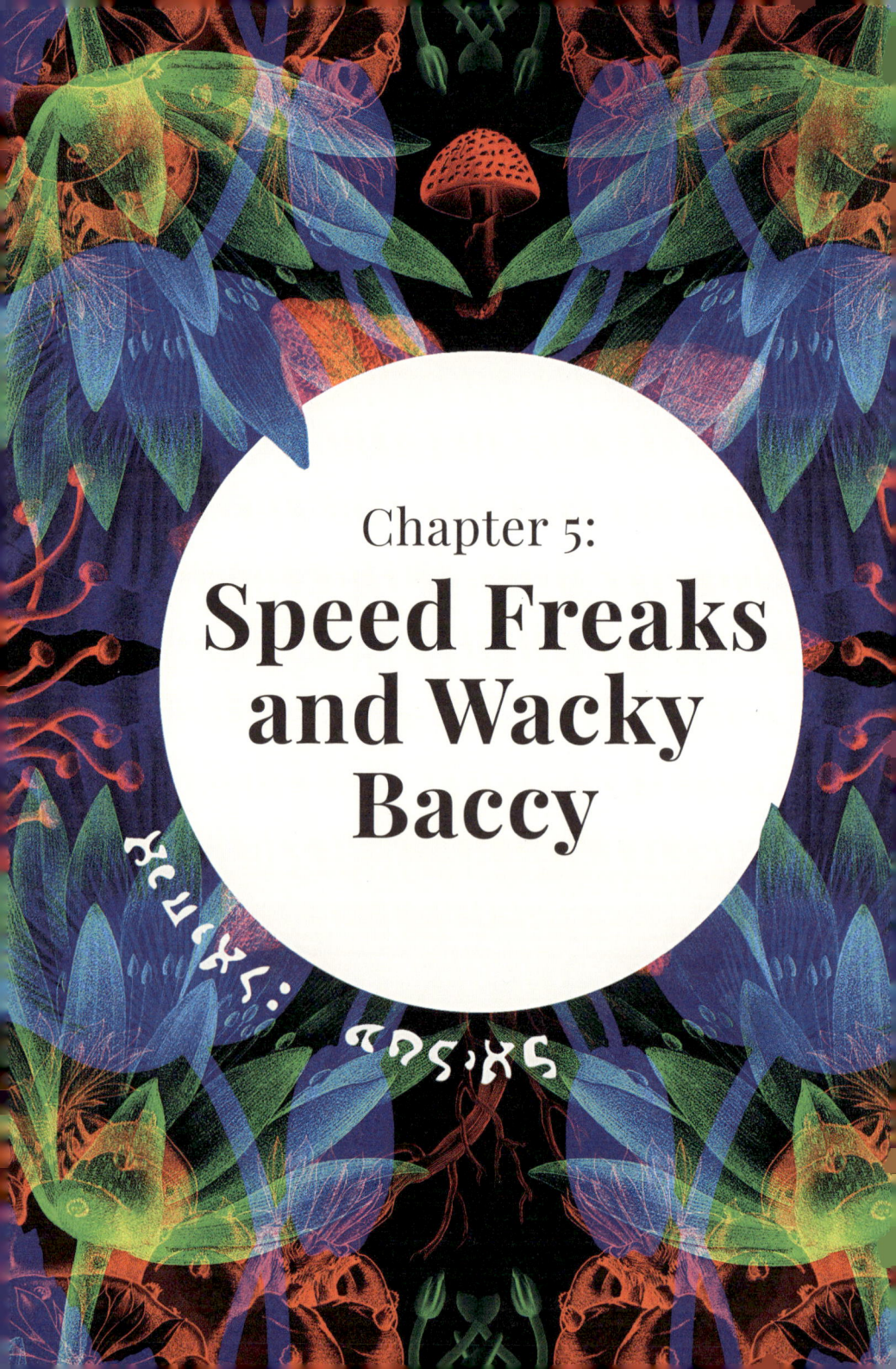

Chapter 5:

Speed Freaks and Wacky Baccy

Some of the world's most widely used "social" drugs are also the most complex. After several millennia no one can quite decide whether cannabis is friend or foe, and while the drug commonly known as speed is amphetamine, the product of a chemistry lab, it has "friends" in nature, including khat, the Middle Eastern favourite. Ecstasy aka MDMA also has a wild chum or two; sprinkle of nutmeg, anyone?

Cannabis
Cannabis sativa

In Hindu mythology the gods and demons joined forces to churn the milk ocean, creating *amrita*, the immortal drink of the gods. Some of the nectar dripped from heaven and wherever it landed on Earth, cannabis sprouted.

The great god Shiva might take issue with that story. While cannabis was included in the *amrita* recipe, some say the blue god himself brought the plant down from the Himalya mountains, for the delight of humans, lending them courage and heightened sexual desire. In yet another story the demons tried to steal the *amrita*. The gods won the epic battle that followed and named its famous ingredient *Vijaya* (Victory).

Such an upbeat story may sound strange in a world that, in the twentieth century, came to revile the plant, giving it a million nicknames – weed, marijuana, pot, grass, skunk, dope, reefer, hash, etc. – few of which sound anything like as optimistic as *victory*. Cannabis has seen its fair share of spins of the wheel of fortune, and it appears to be turning once more.

The Cannabaceae family of plants is fairly small, though one of them is the (non-psychoactive) hops (see p. 59), which gives the bitterness to beer and a whole new meaning to the slang term "hophead".

All parts of the cannabis plant may be useful – the leaves and flower buds as a medicine and narcotic, the seeds for food and lamp oil, and hemp fibre for anything from paper and fishing nets to sails and rope.

The ancients certainly knew about the plant's psychoactive properties. Shennong, the legendary Chinese emperor whose name means "Divine Farmer", suggested that, taken to excess, the fruit will result in seeing demons but over a long period it would allow one to communicate with the spirits. It seems to have been used by Zoroastrian and Mongolian shamans, and the Graeco-Roman physician Galen suggested it was sometimes used at parties to induce hilarity, but hemp was just too useful to overtake other intoxicants.

Historically, the ancient Egyptians used cannabis for eye infections, the Chinese for gout, rheumatism and malaria. Dioscorides's *Materia Medica*, from 70 CE, notes the plant's anti-inflammatory qualities.

England's King Henry VIII encouraged hemp-growing: to build a navy, he needed sails and rope. His daughter Elizabeth I, faced with the Spanish Armada, needed even more, but during the rule of her successor, James VI and I, the industry shifted to plantations in the American colonies, powered by an enslaved workforce. Perhaps it is unsurprising that early drafts of the Declaration of Independence were written on hemp paper.

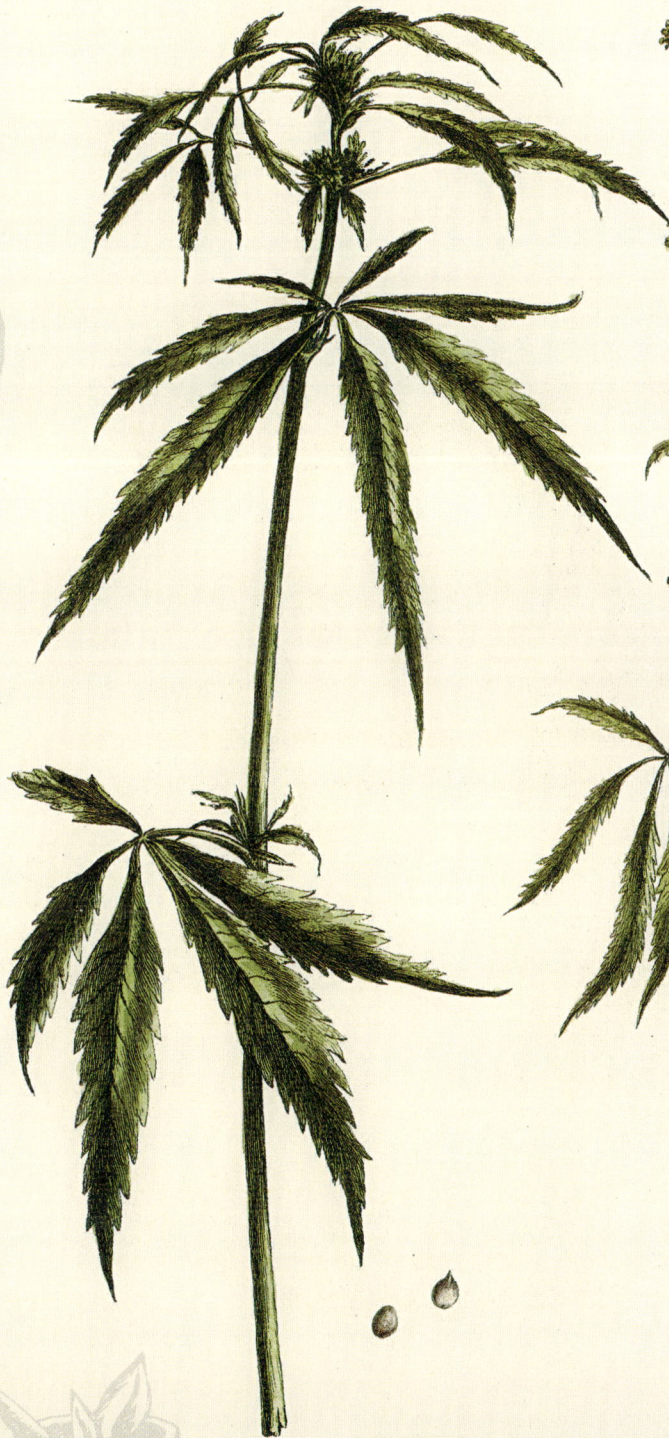

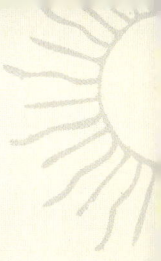

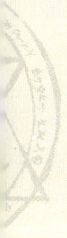

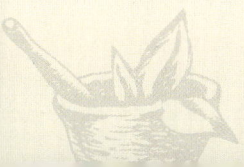

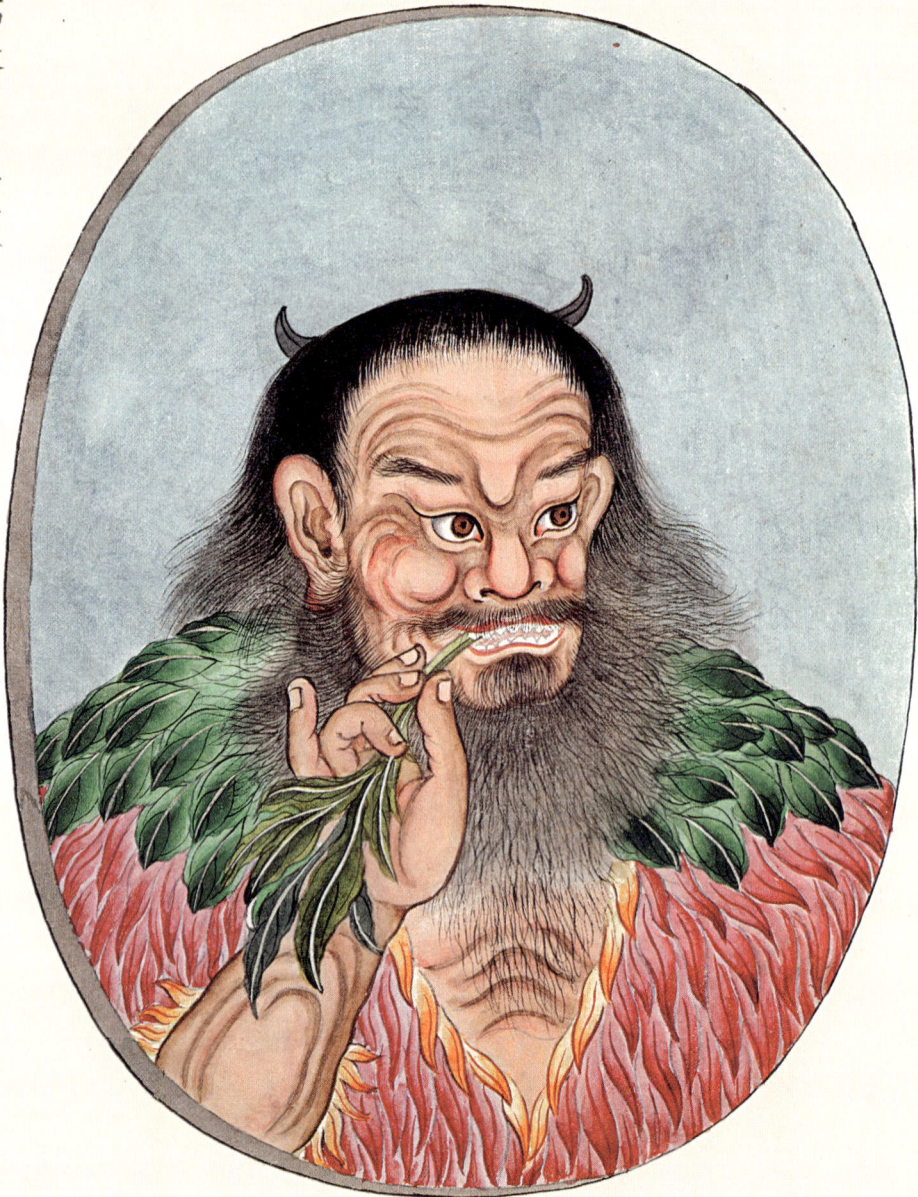

仰惟神農
植藝五穀
以化民育
慮及夭傷
斯民有生
後嘗艸木

Whatever the uses of hemp, cannabis's other, more "cerebral" nature is never far away. It may appear as small wads of dried flower buds; as the brown goo of hashish, made from the plant's resin glands; as an oil, to be inhaled from a heated surface; or even as "green dragon", one of several tinctures extracted from soaked flower buds. It has been eaten, perhaps as "pot brownies", "weed gummies" or "space cakes"; some may miss the romance of the "Arabian Gunjah of Enchantment, the Exhiliratia from Arabia", a late nineteenth-century "hasheesh candy" all the way from exotic Boston, Massachusetts. It has been smoked as a joint (a giant, self-rolled cigarette), bubbled through a bong (water pipe) or slapped on as a patch. The newest kid in groove-town is the electronic "weed vape", which eliminates the pungent smell.

Perceptions of reality may be changed by cannabis, including feelings of euphoria and extreme relaxation where all sensations can be multiplied. Some experience an increased sense of creativity and wonder, where even the most mundane things assume cosmic profundity. On a less exciting side, users often experience dry mouth, dizziness, vomiting, red eyes, increased heart rate and ravenous hunger: the notorious "munchies". Less fun, still, it can lead to anxiety and paranoia. Extended use may manifest in classic "stoner" symptoms: depression, slowness of thought, fatigue and memory problems, definitively portrayed by Jeff Bridges as The Dude in *The Big Lebowski* (1998).

Cannabis is frowned on by most Muslim societies but remains popular with Sufism, which considers it sacred, a manifestation of divine blessing, another way to experience the wonder of creation. For Hindus, the consumption of *bhang* – anything edible made from the plant – it is believed to deter evil. *Bhang* is enjoyed at festivals as a vessel of prayer and meditation, often led by Sadhus, itinerant holy men.

The religion most closely associated with cannabis is Rastafarianism, mainly practised by diasporic Africans of the Caribbean. Begun in the 1930s, the movement suggests that Rastas (followers) await their return to Zion after being tested by God via the horrors of slavery.

Rastas believe that the original Tree of Life was cannabis, and that smoking ganja, sometimes from a chalice (pipe), allows them to meditate with Jah (God).

From a relatively laissez-faire approach in the early twentieth century, concern grew about the effects of cannabis consumption and morphed into a kind of hysteria as it gained a reputation as a party drug for anyone from jazz musicians and flappers to beatniks and then nice young college kids. It was made illegal in the UK in 1928 and, after years of restriction, banned in the USA in 1937, but that only seemed to fuel the plant's mystical allure. Cannabis became a poster drug for the 1960s' dropout counterculture, and it still carries an element of rebellion. Even the leaf is iconic, its image plastered over T-shirts, jewellery and teenagers' bedroom

Opposite The legendary emperor Shen-Nung, who is often pictured with a cannabis leaf in his mouth.

walls. Bill Clinton's admission to experimenting with the drug as a student in 1992 (while probably truthfully claiming never to have inhaled; he ate hash brownies) added a bad-boy frisson to his presidential candidacy.

Yet the tide is turning for this complex chameleon, which has been so many things to so many people. While much research has been done on cannabidiol (CBD), a compound found in cannabis, a lot of its potential beneficial effects are not completely confirmed, but the sheer weight of anecdotal evidence is shifting public opinion. Considered to carry fewer side effects than opioid drugs such as morphine, cannabis has been welcomed by some people suffering certain types of chronic pain, while cannabinoids and their

derivatives are of interest for use in conditions such as multiple sclerosis and epilepsy. The synthetic cannabinoid nabilone is used to help reduce nausea for people undergoing chemotherapy. Cannabis is also being investigated for the management of conditions including post-traumatic stress disorder.

With so much research being undertaken, a growing number of countries are legalizing medicinal cannabis. Fewer are happy to see it easily available for recreational purposes. While some, such as Canada, Germany and Thailand, have decided they are better off regulating and taxing the supply, others have merely decriminalized the plant. Most remain firmly in the "illegal" camp. Punishments range from a slap on the metaphorical wrist to (extremely rare) mandatory execution.

Opposite A poster for *Reefer Madness*, an anti-drugs exploitation film dealing with the pitfalls of smoking marijuana.

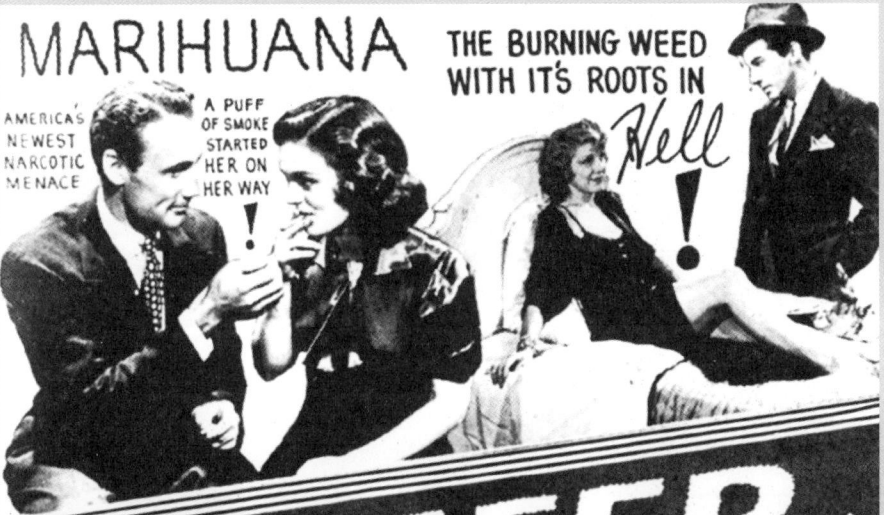

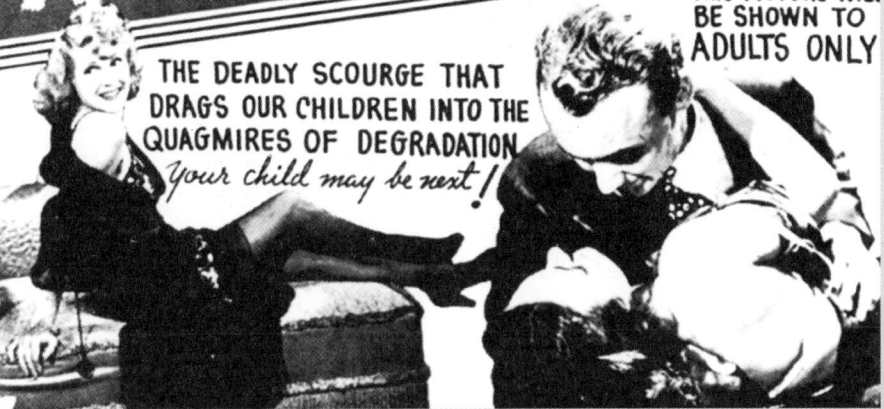

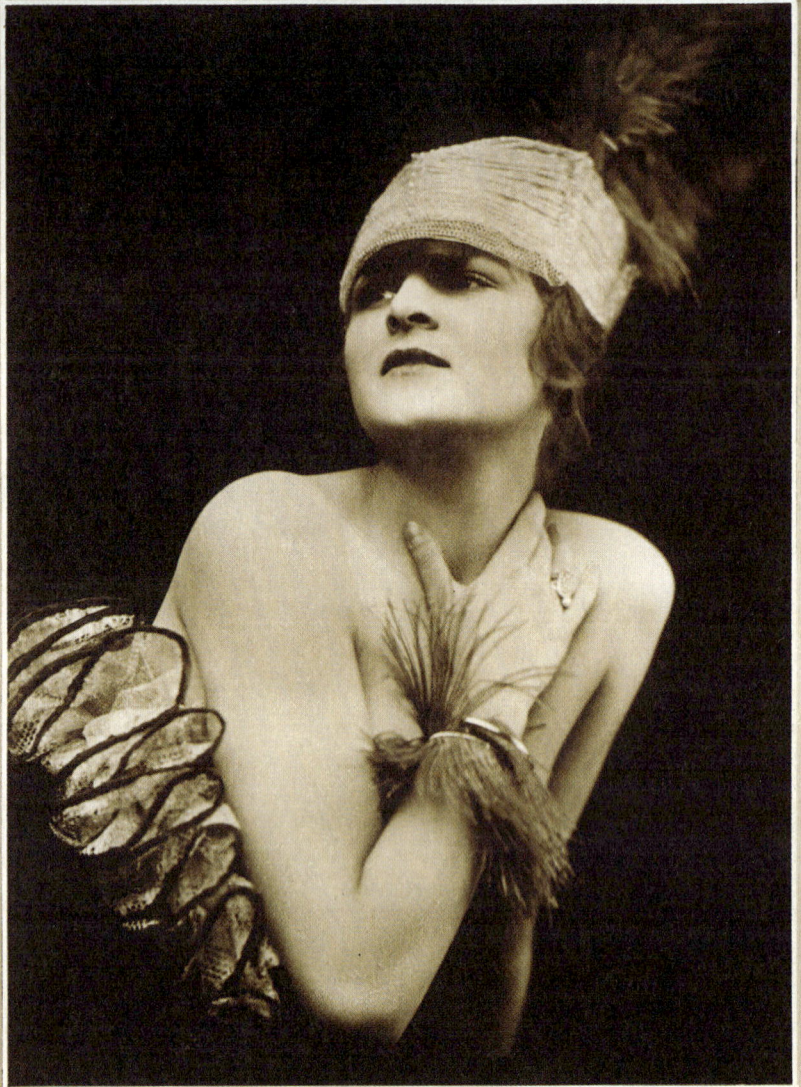

Bildnis von Anny Eberth, Berlin.

ANITA BERBER

If You're a Viper:
Drugs in the 1920s and '30s

The sky is high and so am I...

The war to end all wars was over. The generation blinking into the harsh daylight of the 1920s was battered, bruised and determined to forget.

The bright young people of London's party scene threw themselves into a desperate round of hedonistic alcohol and drug-fuelled fancy dress balls, country house parties and scavenger hunts. Much of the bohemian styling – flapper-style short skirts, cropped hair, fast cars and jazz – was indulged by Britain's aristocratic youth, but in the picture-houses "It Girl" Clara Bow was proving that even a shopgirl could have fun if she was plucky enough. They were sure having crazy times across the pond...

Things weren't quite as much fun in the United States as they looked, though. Between 1920 and 1933, Prohibition laws banned the production, transportation and sale of alcohol. Not that it stopped anyone. Underground speakeasies served bootleg liquor alongside a range of other substances. Hallucinogens were not used widely, but cannabis, cocaine and opiates were and many of the jazz musicians playing in such establishments used them all, hotly pursued by the authorities. Some preferred to skip town altogether.

In Paris, the *Années folles* (crazy years) were in full swing. Art deco, Dada, surrealism and all manner of other isms burned bright in a dazzling night scene, a haven for Black musicians facing racism at home. Artist René Gaillard summed up the scene in a famous poster for the 1925 play *Cocaine*: featuring a green goblin, red-dressed flapper, bespectacled intellectual, jazz saxophonist, the Moulin Rouge nightclub and the Sacré-Coeur Basilica.

Germany had been on the wrong side of the Versailles Treaty. The Kaiser was gone, and the Weimar Republic that replaced him was weak. There was little left to do but party. The Berlin cabaret scene was a heady cocktail of sexual liberation, debauchery and Peruvian cocaine. Other drugs were also freely available; users just blended in with the war veterans who had been prescribed morphine and heroin for their chronic pain, physical and mental.

Anita Berber was the wildest cat in the wildest city on earth. Her "exotic" dance routines had names like "Cocaine" and "Morphium", but these were only two of the substances she might ingest in a day. It was said she started out with a breakfast bowl of chloroform and ether, stirred with a white rose, getting her fibre from its petals, before moving on to everything else available. Incredibly, in 1928, at the age of 29, Berber decided to get clean. She even managed it. Alas, a few months later, she died anyway, from tuberculosis.

It was a wake-up call, but no one heard it. Berlin's *Glückliche Zwanziger* (Happy Twenties) roared on, even as the shirts outside the dance halls turned ever more brown.

Opposite Anita Berber's penchant for drugs, decadence and self destruction made her infamous.

Morning glory

Ipomoea

A vast, entwined genus within the even bigger Convolvulaceae family, *Ipomoea* contains more than 600 species that snake their way around the world causing delight, dismay and not a small amount of confusion.

Whether delighted in by gardeners as showy ornamental scramblers such as *Ipomoea purpurea*, spread across the South Pacific islands as a "canoe plant" to feed the world with sweet potato (*I. batatas*) or used in root form as "John the Conquerer" (*I. purga*) in African American Hoodoo "mojo bags", the uses are myriad. The Olmec people of Mesoamerica even treated latex from *Castilla elastica* with *I. alba* to make bouncing balls three thousand years before vulcanisation was invented by the Global North. Only a few *Ipomoea* species are known to contain psychoactive alkaloids but they are, perhaps, most confusing of all.

Even the names are a puzzle. *Ipomoea* is rooted in the ancient Greek for woodworm, and the species names sometimes describe contradictory attributes. *Ipomoea violacea* (beach or sea moonflower), for example, does not have the purple flower that *violacea* suggests but is pure white. Its small round seeds may contain lysergic acid derivatives and ergometrine, giving it LSD-like properties, though it needs to be consumed in large quantities to gain similar psychedelic effects. It's often confused with *I. tricolor* (heavenly blue), which contains similar psychoactive compounds. Side effects from consuming *Ipomoea* can include hallucination, nausea and diarrhoea.

The famous medicinal "Ololiuhqui", which was first championed, then suppressed, by Spanish colonists in Mexico may refer to several plants, but early illustrations suggest some kind of morning glory. Richard Evans Schultes suggested the psychoactive Christmas vine, *I. corymbosa*, as the most likely candidate, though he also mentioned *I. violacea* as a sacred hallucinogenic among certain Mexican communities and *I. carnea*, sometimes used in South America. Schultes sent some seeds of *I. corymbosa* to Albert Hofmann, the inventor of LSD, who discovered lysergic acid compounds, usually found in ergot fungus. The plant's chemical make-up is still not fully understood.

Morning glory's short-lived, funnel-shaped flowers seem to represent the brevity of life – in Japan it is a symbol of mortality.

Ipomoea's relative, Hawaiian baby woodrose (*Argyreia nervosa*), is another puzzle, being neither a rose nor from Hawaii, but it does contain similar, highly potent psychedelic ergoline alkaloids. Native to India, *A. nervosa* has been used in Ayurvedic medicine for centuries, but its only known use as an entheogen was, until the 1960s, in Nepal.

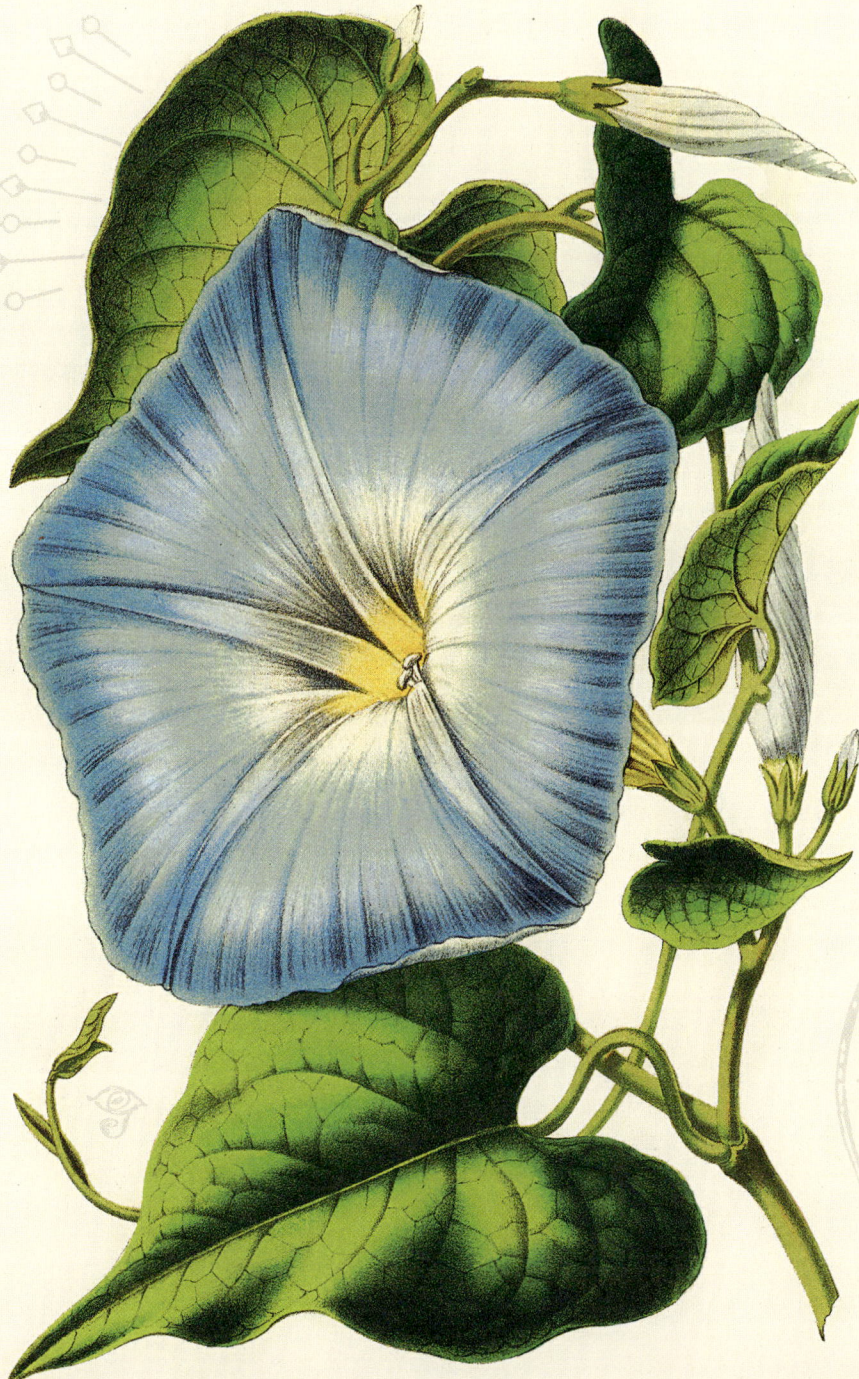

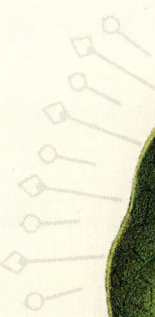

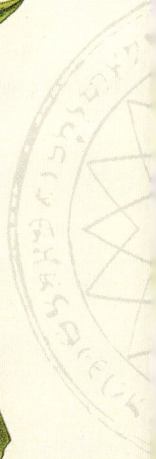

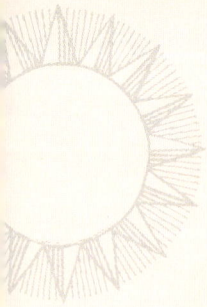

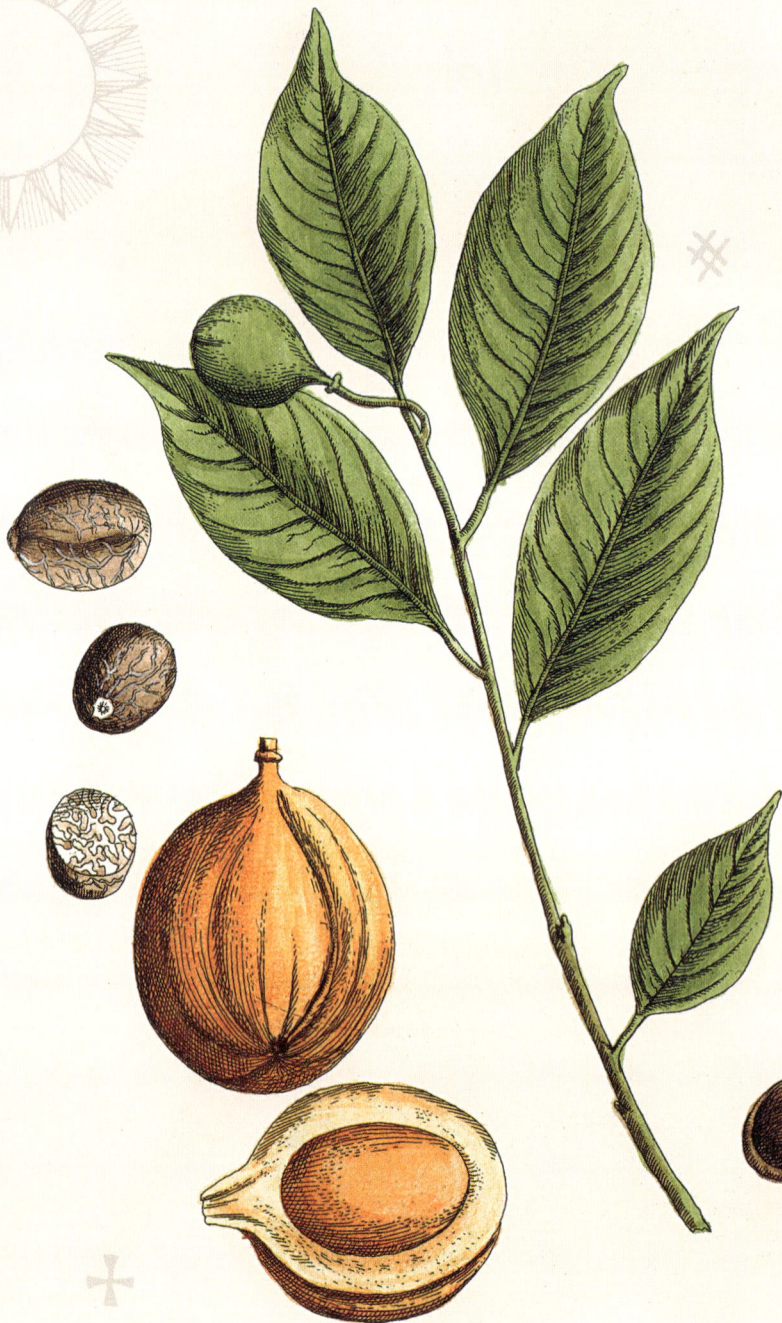

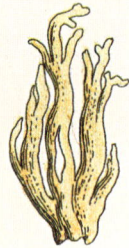

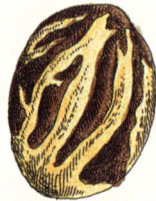

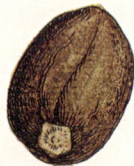

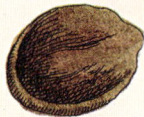

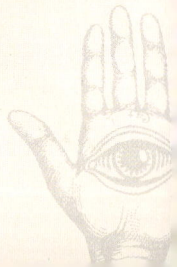

Nutmeg

Myristica fragrans

Malcolm X's 1965 autobiography pulls no punches about his early, hellish experiences in Charleston State Prison. Seeking any kind of relief, he turned to nutmeg.

He wrote: "Stirred into a glass of cold water, a penny matchbox full of nutmeg had the kick of three or four reefers." Jailhouse reefers can't have been very strong. Nutmeg contains myristicin, which the tree may produce as a natural insecticide, but considerable quantities are needed to gain any kind of high. Yet this is a spice over which countries have been lost and regimes toppled.

This handsome, evergreen tree is indigenous to the Banda Islands in the Moluccas (Spice Islands) of Indonesia. Nutmeg seed and its desiccated *aril* (casing) appears in Hindu Vedas composed between 1500 and 1000 BCE considered as useful against colds, halitosis and digestive complaints. It was equally prized when it reached Europe, sometime around the sixth century. Alongside its fragrance, flavour and usefulness in medicine, it has also long been known for its psychoactive effects. The Benedictine abbess Hildegard of Bingen used nutmeg in her famous "cookies of joy", writing in 1157 that the spice would open the heart, clear judgement and create a good disposition. Legends grew. Carrying a small bag of nutmeg was believed to ward off plague, prevent broken bones and generally repel evil.

Local traders did not stand a chance when the Portuguese arrived on the islands, starting a chain of violence as various European powers fought to monopolize the only place where *Myristica fragrans* grew. The Portuguese were ousted by the Dutch and, in 1667, the British gave up their small claim on the Banda Islands in return for a swampy area on the east coast of America they eventually renamed Manhattan, meanwhile cannily planting smuggled *Myristica fragrans* seeds elsewhere – presumably leaving the Dutch wondering why they hadn't thought of that one themselves.

Ingesting large amounts of fresh seed, usually ground into some kind of drink, may (eventually) produce weak hallucinations, bright colours, euphoria and a sense of disconnection that some have likened to the effects of marijuana, but the high dosage has some unpleasant consequences. Convulsions, dry mouth, palpitations, nausea and diarrhoea are often followed by severe headaches. That has not stopped people trying. Saxophonist Charlie Parker and writer William S. Burroughs both dabbled in nutmeg, and thanks to another compound present in the seed, safrole, it is sometimes used in the street drug ecstasy.

Khat

Catha edulis

In Kenya, if someone finds a statement hard to believe. they may say: *"hio ni stori ya jaba"*, implying it is a story "of the streets", of *Jaba*, one of the many names for the nation's favourite narcotic.

Once chewed by the elderly to help them pray, an estimated three quarters of Yemeni and Somali men chew khat daily. This was traditionally a male pastime, though women and even children now use khat across East Africa and the Middle East. Arguments rage over its status: revered cultural tradition or public health scourge?

A flowering plant from the Celastraceae (staff-vine) family, *Catha edulis* produces dark, glossy leaves that are usually chewed, with leaves gradually added until the quid fills the cheeks. Some people smoke the leaves or make an infusion, giving the brew another range of names: Abyssinian, Somalian, Arabian and Bushman's Teas. In Israel it is known as *gat*. Whatever its name, khat is centuries old.

Khat contains the alkaloid cathinone, an amphetamine-like stimulant and hunger suppressant, making it popular with long-distance lorry drivers. Users may experience dilated pupils and increased heart rate and blood pressure. Prolonged use can cause aggression, dizziness, paranoia, psychosis, depression and cardiovascular disorders. Also associated with khat are gastrointestinal tumours and oral cancers, though these may be the result of chemical fertilizers used to cultivate the plant. Long-

term users may also suffer tooth decay, constipation, ulcers and a diminished sex drive.

With such side effects, it may seem surprising so many partake, but the drug's mildly euphoric sensations, together with its social opportunities and traditional values, provide a profound sense of escape. Critics in Somalia have labelled it the opium of the people.

Ethiopian legend tells us that *merkhana* was a word invented by Sufi imams to describe a state of mind enabling a union with God through consuming khat. Today the term is used more generally for a khat high. Seeking *merkhana* has engendered a powerful cash-crop economy. Cultivation involves huge areas of land and vast amounts of irrigation, sometimes leaving communities without running water.

The leaves rapidly lose potency after harvesting, creating a daily race to sell and buy the freshest product. This may be the reason that khat has never caught on elsewhere. When fifteenth-century European traders were sampling coffee, khat was equally popular in the Arabian port of Mocha. Beans were less perishable and easier to transport, so the world became a planet of coffee drinkers.

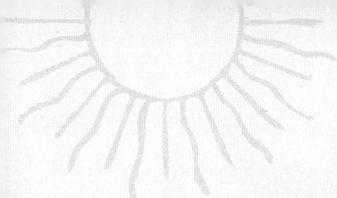

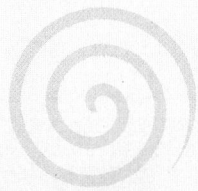

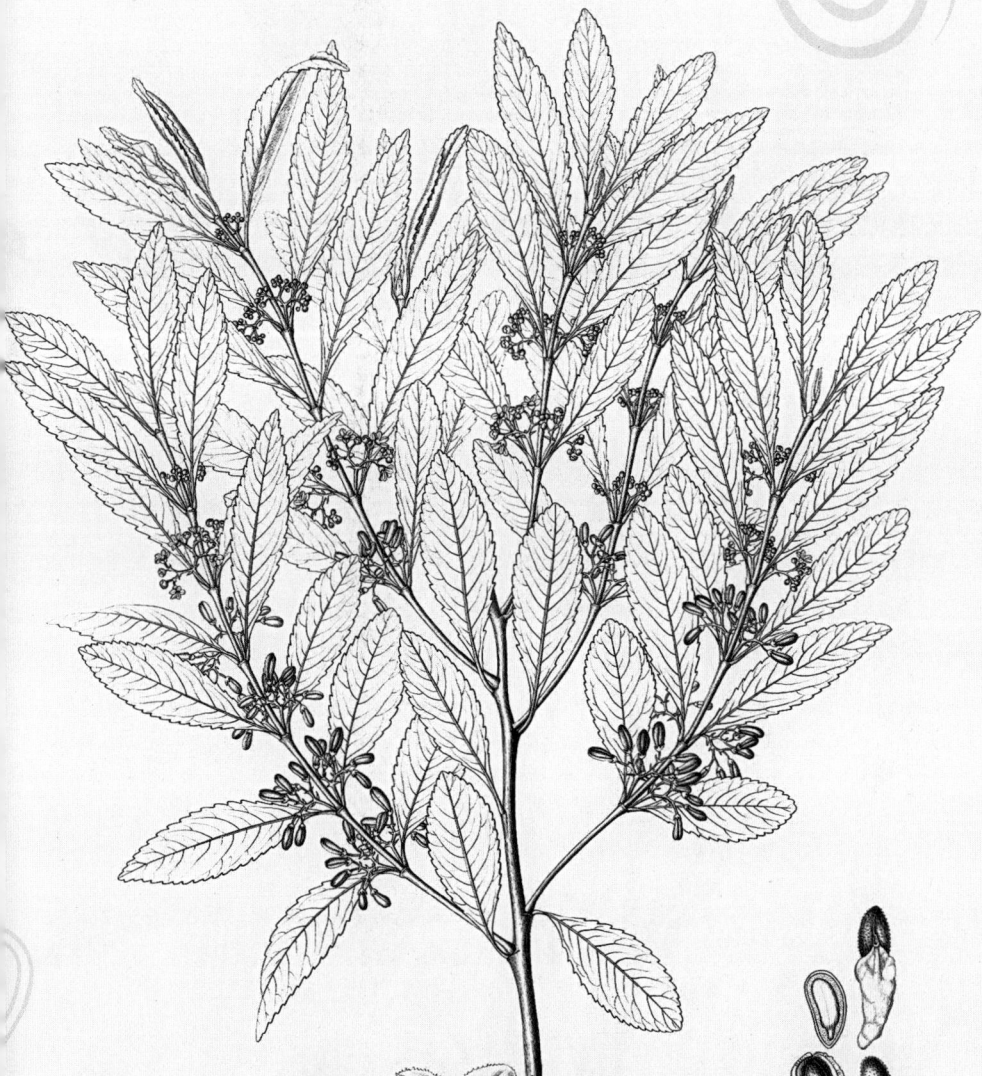

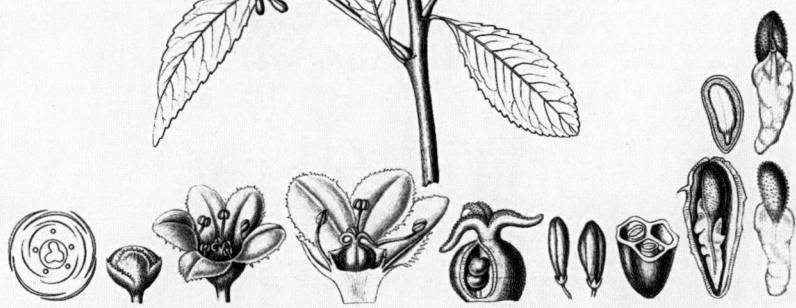

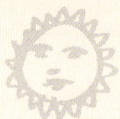

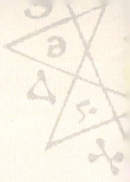

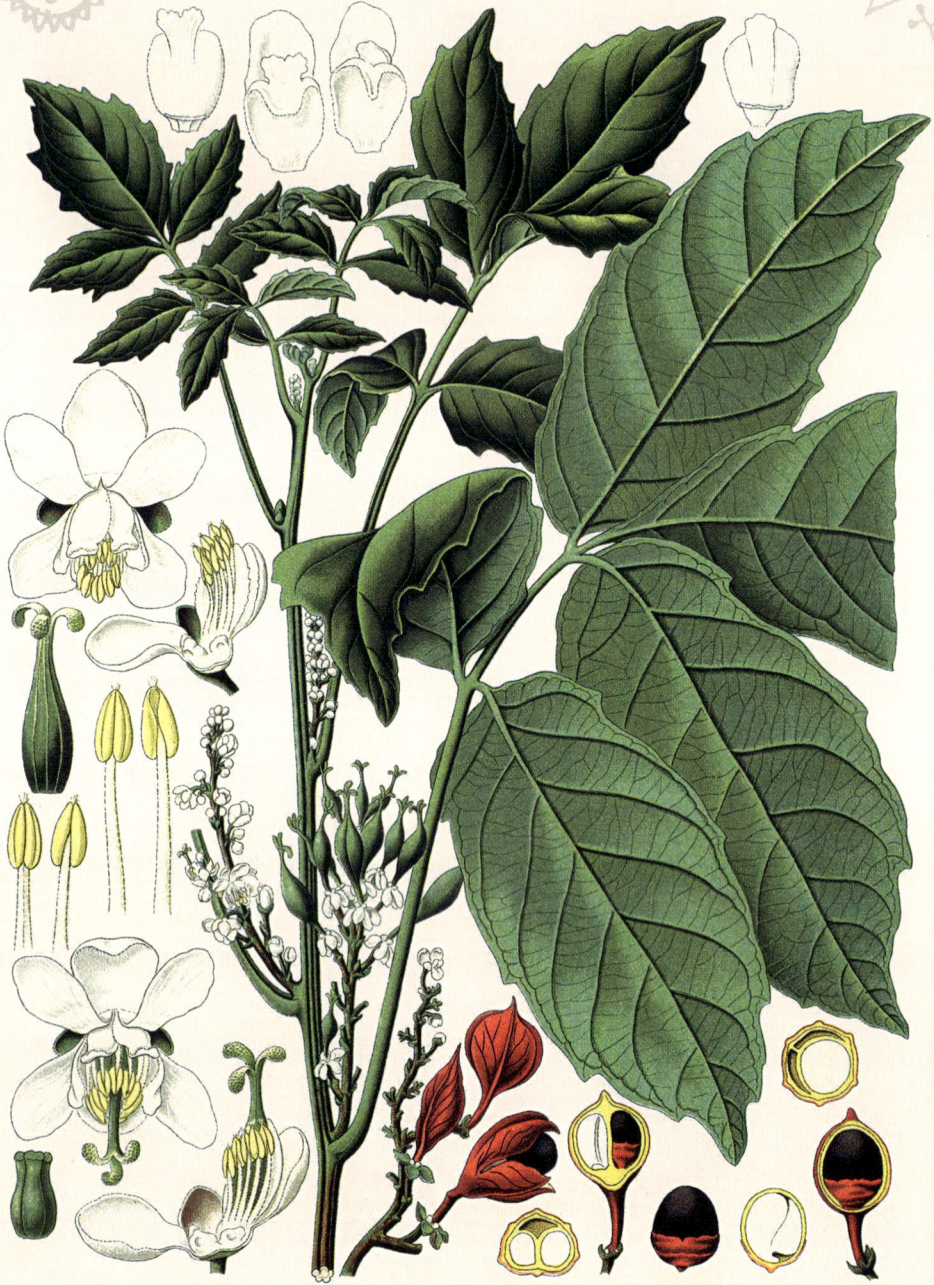

Guarana

Paullinia cupana

Deep in the Amazonian rainforest, something is watching.
A cluster of scarlet-lidded eyes, their whites brilliant and clear,
their pupils black, following your every move.

Every year Brazilian people drink upwards of 400 million litres of Guaraná Antártica, an energizing soft drink made from guarana, a climbing plant from the soapberry (Sapindaceae) family. Perhaps unsurprisingly, all the legends involving *Paullinia cupana* involve eyes, and although varying in detail, have one grisly theme: the eyes of a murdered child.

Ancient stories from the Guarani people tell of a childless couple, finally granted a beautiful boy by the god Tupã. The child collected fruit from the forest for the entire village and everyone assumed he would grow up to be chief, but Jurapari, the jealous god of darkness, turned himself into a snake and bit the boy. Some say Tupã advised the parents to pluck out their dead child's eyes and plant them, others claim the god did the deed himself. Whichever version is told, the parents' tears watered the strange plant that grew from the grave.

Some expand the tale to involve three siblings, one of whom was seduced by a snake and gave birth to the boy. The woman's brothers, who despised the boy's origins, had him killed. On finding his body, the distraught mother plucked out the child's eyes and planted them. The left grew into the false guarana, the right eye produced the real thing. The woman then buried the rest of the boy's body. Various animals emerged from the grave, which she cursed, until her son was reborn as the first of the Mawé.

Guarana is a sacred plant for the Mawé, bringing good luck and warding off evil spirits. Its seeds are carried as protective amulets, but also, today, as a symbol of cultural identity as the rest of South America wakes up to guarana's powers.

The Mawé still cultivate their own guarana, first drying, then roasting the seeds and grinding them to a powder, which they mix with water to make handy cylindrical batons. A little may be pared away for use as a medicine to combat diarrhoea, fevers or headaches or to repel insects. More often, it is scraped into hot water and sweetened with honey to make earthy-flavoured *çapó*, a beverage considerably higher in caffeine than coffee. Strict cultural rules govern its drinking, including the way the gourd should be passed, and who serves the drink. Most importantly, the bowl should never be fully emptied.

In excess, guarana can have side effects, including insomnia, anxiety, heart palpitations and stomach upsets.

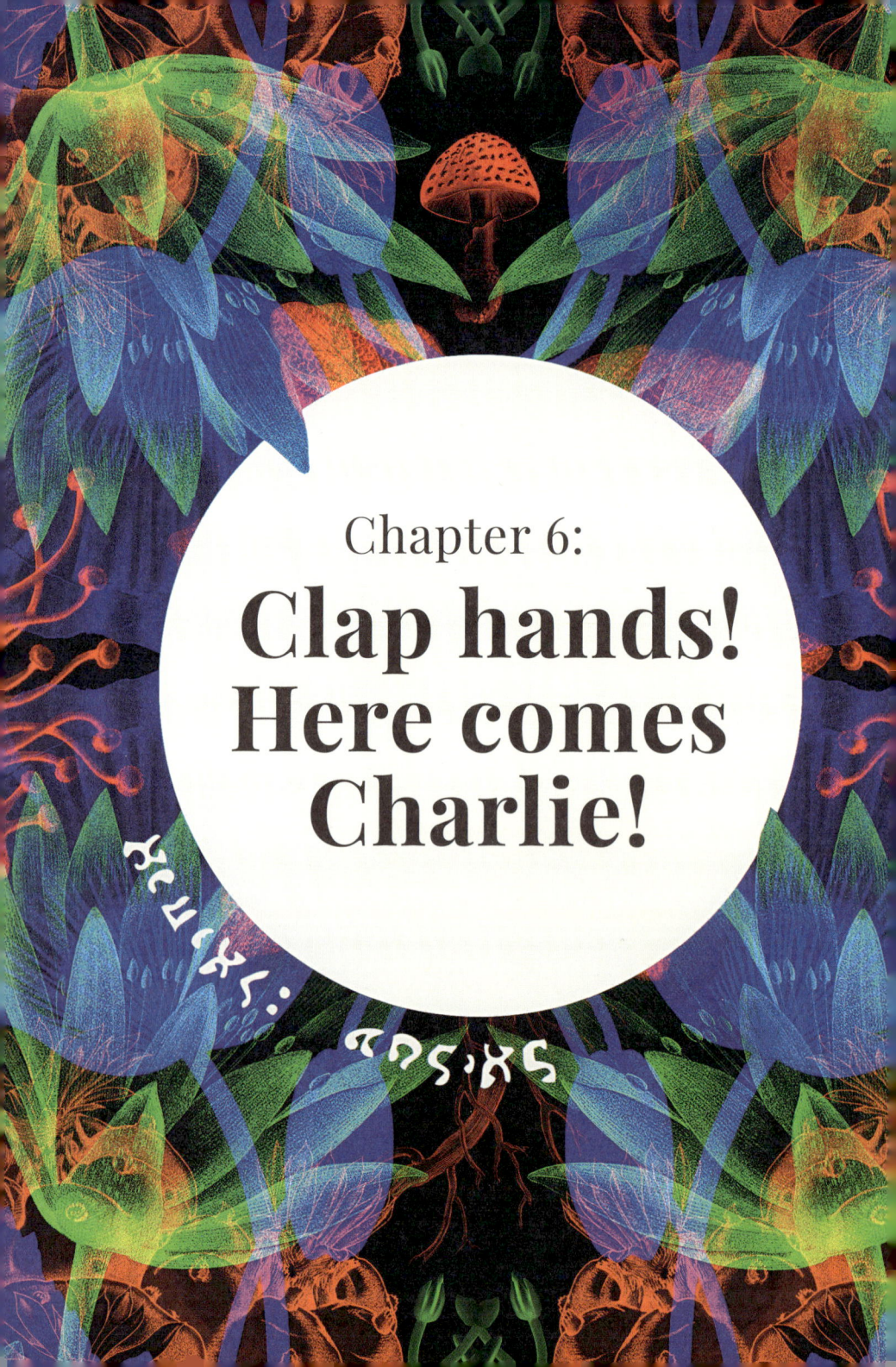

Chapter 6:

Clap hands!
Here comes
Charlie!

Cocaine is an emotive word. In one stereotype, it conjures Hollywood A-listers, rock stars and sharp-suited businessmen in private jets snorting white powder from mirrors through rolled up hundred-dollar bills. In another cliché, out-of-control drug cartels shoot each other across crowded city streets and terrorize entire communities. Both images are crude, cartoon-like exaggerations, but they also carry an element of truth. Neither has much to do with the substance's origins.

Coca

Erythroxylum coca

Mama Coca was famous for her devastating beauty, which roused jealous passions and fighting among young men. The Council of the Wise told the Inca (king) she must be sacrificed for the sake of the empire.

Parts of Mama Coca's body were buried in the gardens of each of her lovers. Small plants began to grow from them, which were named in tribute to her. Not everyone agrees with this story. Some will tell you that *khoka*, which just means "the tree", was the only plant that grew after Khuno, god of snow and thunder, sent a firestorm that devastated the land. Emerging from their shelter caves, people discovered that the leaves could sustain and cheer them, so they named the sacred herb *Pachamama*, after the Earth Goddess.

People of the Andean regions of Peru, Colombia, Brazil, Bolivia, Ecuador, Northern Argentina and Chile have been chewing coca since pre-Inca times — as a mild stimulant; to endure hunger, pain and cold; to alleviate the effects of high-altitude, low-oxygen environments; and as a treatment for any number of ailments. A symbol of cultural and religious identity that links indigenous cultures throughout South America, it is both a part of daily life and a pivotal aspect of indigenous spirituality. Coca is among the major offerings to the Apus, spirits of the mountains, to Inti, god of the sun, and to Pachamama herself.

Archaeological evidence suggests that Peruvian foraging peoples were chewing coca leaves up to 8,000 years ago. Mummies buried with a supply of dried leaves for the afterlife, pottery depictions of "chewers" and decorative masks of faces with a familiar "bulge" in their cheeks bring a human edge to such finds. Coca was so important to the Inca people that only the nobility could chew it outside spiritual use. All that went with the Spanish invasion. After initially denouncing it as satanic, the Catholic Church accepted that giving coca to enslaved gold and silver miners allowed them to work harder, longer and with less sustenance. Taxing it even produced extra income.

Coca contains tropane alkaloids, notably cocaine and cinnamylcocaine, in addition to other substances including an essential oil. Chewing (or to be more precise, sucking) coca is a national pastime, including much everyday ritual. Someone's *chuspa* or *huallqepo* (coca leaf bag) may explain much about them. Supposedly simple, these pieces of intricately woven fabric stitched up the sides were once used by nobility and only royalty had fringing, but they have spread in popularity. Patterns, textiles, beads, tassels and other ornamentation indicate someone's profession and status. An accompanying *poporo* contains the lime substance (once bone or seashells,

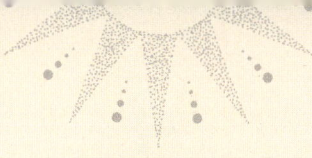

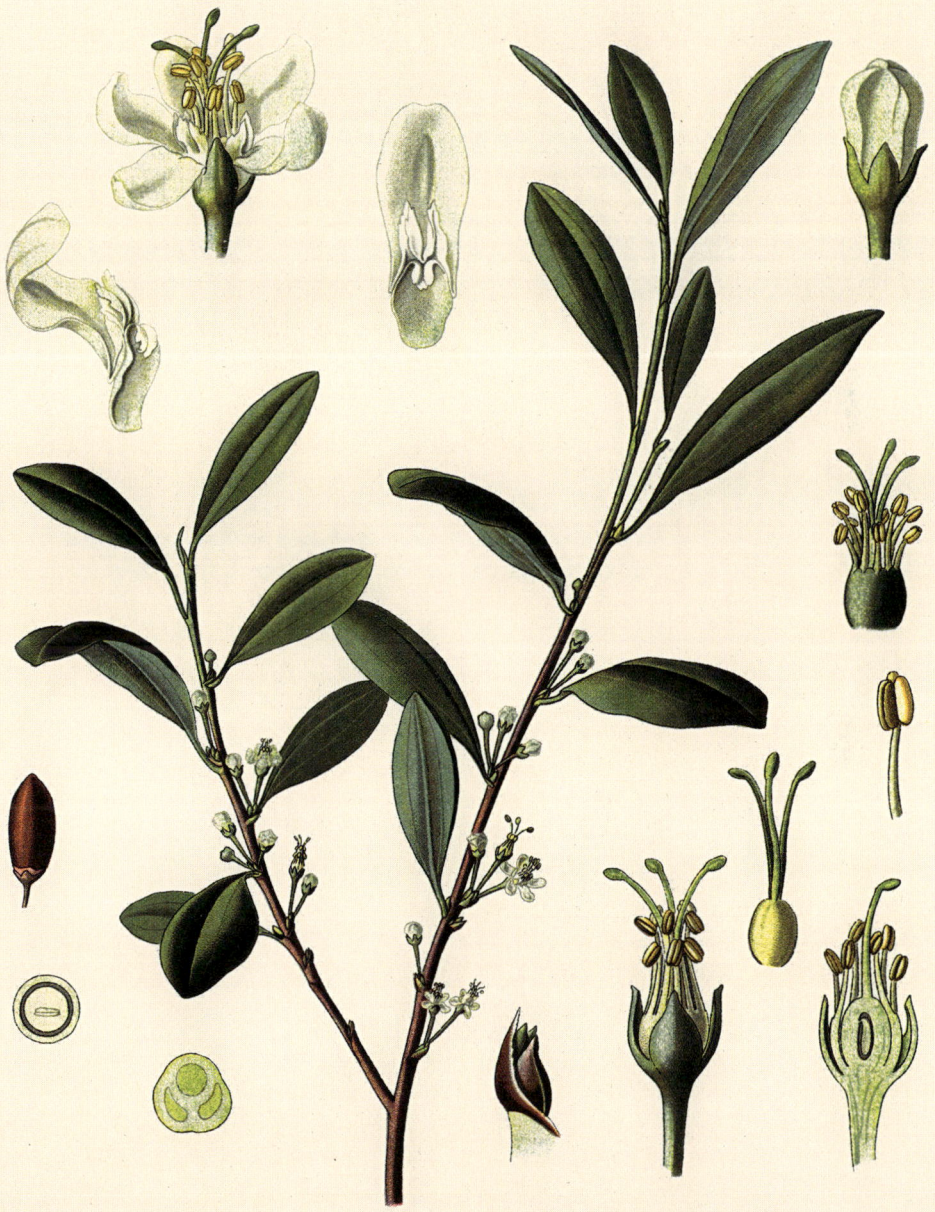

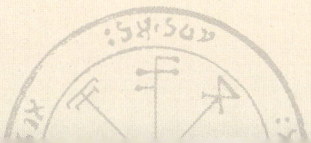

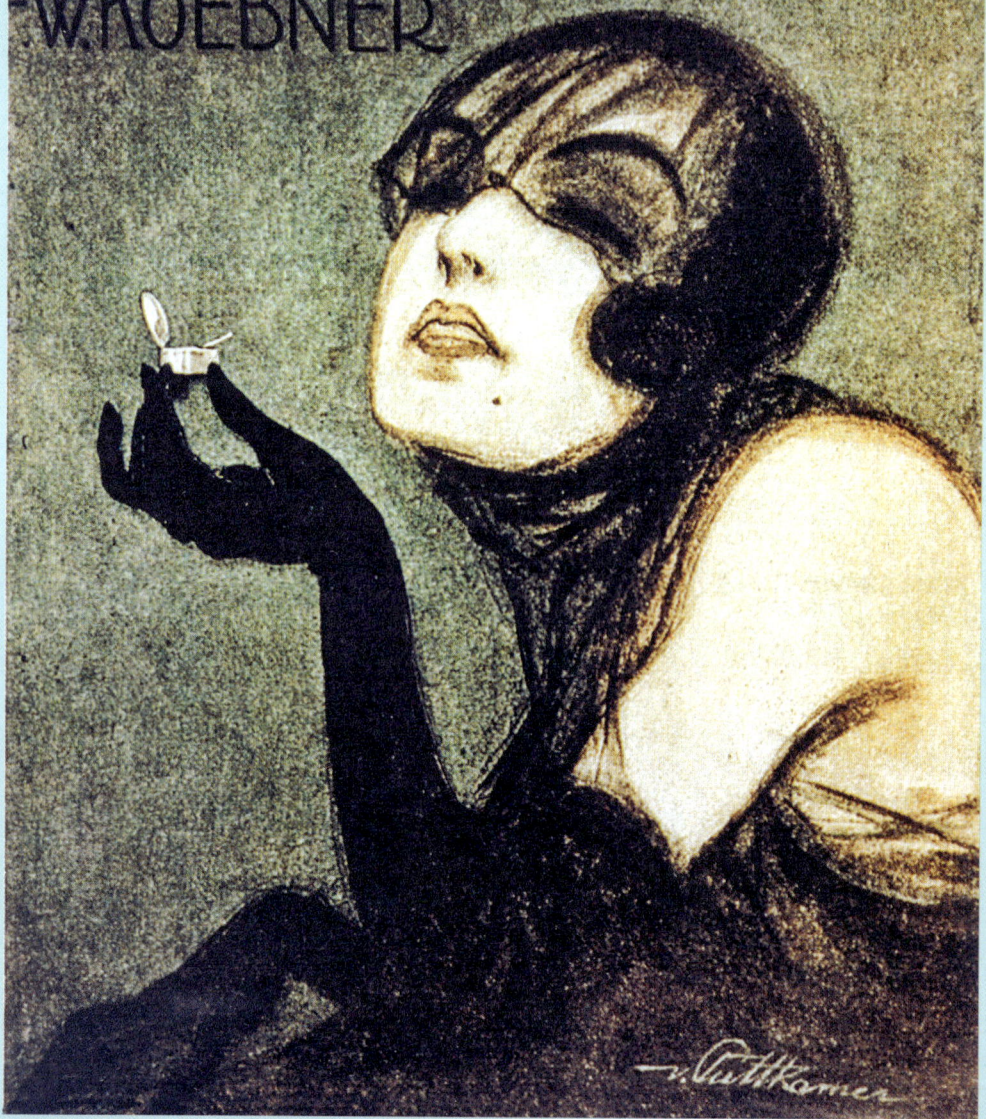

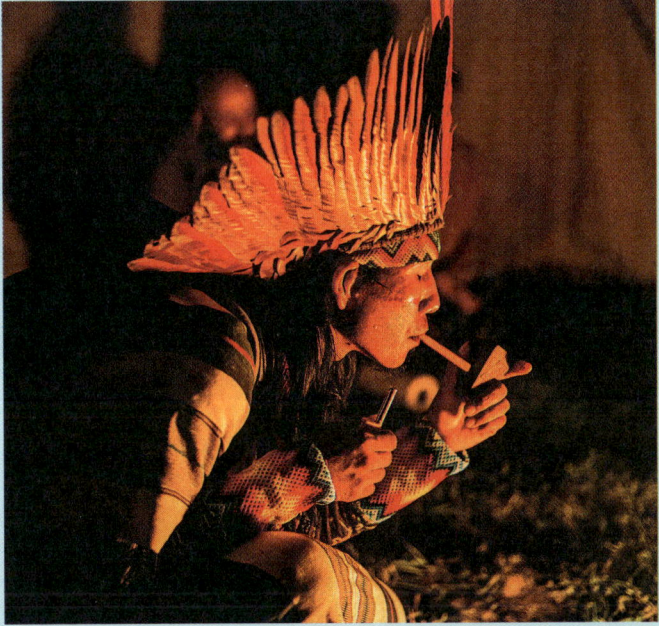

Right A shaman smokes a pipe to begin a ritual at Pachamama festival, where they hold ayahuasca, rapé, temezcal and peyote ceremonies.

Opposite A Berlin poster representing the new fashion for taking drugs, here showing a woman taking cocaine.

now mainly bicarbonate of soda) that activates the leaf. These, too, are often elaborate. In some cultures – Kogi, for example – young men are given a *poporo* when they reach adulthood.

While chewing can be a solo activity or part of a spiritual ceremony, in some communities, including Quechua, it is also a social ritual, especially when welcoming guests. Someone will select three of their best leaves, fan them between their thumb and forefinger, blow gently across them as an act of gratitude to Pachamama, then pass them to a friend as an invitation to chew. The recipient receives them with both palms opened together.

Leaves are prepared for chewing by removing the tough midrib. They are then placed in the side of the mouth and slowly added to until a quid forms, which will be chewed for between 30 and 90 minutes before the juice is swallowed and the quid spat out. The taste is initially bitter, gradually easing to a grassy flavour.

After about 10 minutes the mouth becomes numb; this is the same numbness that inspired the design of certain anaesthetics in Western medicine, which are based on cocaine. In traditional medicine where coca is indigenous, women are sometimes advised to chew coca during childbirth to relieve the pain and hasten the arrival of the baby, but coca's numbing effects are not the only reasons people use it medicinally. It is alleged to alleviate complaints as wide-ranging as constipation, asthma, malaria and the pangs of love.

Given the Catholic Church's stance in previous centuries, it is a curious twist that Pope Francis, on being offered coca tea to stave off altitude sickness on a papal visit to Bolivia in 2015, asked to chew coca leaves as well. It is unclear whether he did, but as an Argentinian-born South American, his request remains a powerful symbol for a continent that sees nothing wrong with the plant, other than what other parts of the world have done with it.

Cocaine

In 1860 the German chemist Albert Niemann isolated a
chemical from the coca leaf, which he named cocaine.
At first no one was really sure what to do with it.

The new substance's numbing effects were quickly discovered and experiments showed interesting anaesthetic properties, but because the purity was inconsistent, so were the results. The race to find cocaine's true purpose had begun.

In the early 1880s Sigmund Freud and his close friend Karl Koller were at medical school in Vienna, both hoping to make their names in some field or other. In 1884, at great expense, Freud bought a gram of cocaine, with the intention of trying to help another friend who had become addicted to morphine. He shared the cocaine with Koller too, then spent some time practising on himself before coming up with a seminal publication, *Über Coca*, where he suggested it as a substance to treat addiction. Unfortunately, although he suggested the drug to be taken orally, most addicts injected it and within months were hooked on both morphine and cocaine.

Freud also mentioned cocaine might work as an anaesthetic, though he had not conducted any deep research into the matter. It was Koller who followed up the idea after a friend remarked it made his tongue numb. His paper, presented a few months after *Über Coca* was published, began the widespread use of cocaine in ophthalmic surgery – and ended Koller's friendship with Freud, who had to look elsewhere for fame.

Along with being useful as a local anaesthetic, cocaine was sold openly in both Europe and the United States as a general tonic and an elixir against pretty much any complaint, from furred tongue to flatulence. It was even sold as a tooth whitener. Slowly, the white powder gained a reputation as a glamorous recreational substance.

Whatever its nickname – blow, coke, snow, dust, nose candy, Charlie; the list goes on – cocaine enters the bloodstream very quickly, giving an instantaneous high. It lasts only a short time, inducing users to crave more. Crack cocaine, cooked with baking soda and crackling as it is heated, is either snorted, smoked or injected, making the hit stronger, more intense and even more addictive.

Cocaine is illegal in most countries, which has led to a thriving and brutal black market, but it is important to remember one thing: cocaine and its attendant problems were developed in Europe and exported back to South America. Coca barons may operate from South America, but their raison d'être lies with the Global North, not the indigenous people who have revered the coca plant for millennia.

Opposite A movie poster for *Cocaine: The Thrill That Kills* in the 1940s. Directed by Giorgio Bianchi, the film follows a cocaine trafficker who attempts to prove his son innocent in a murder case.

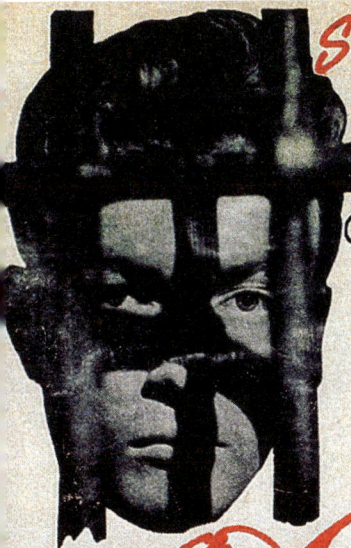

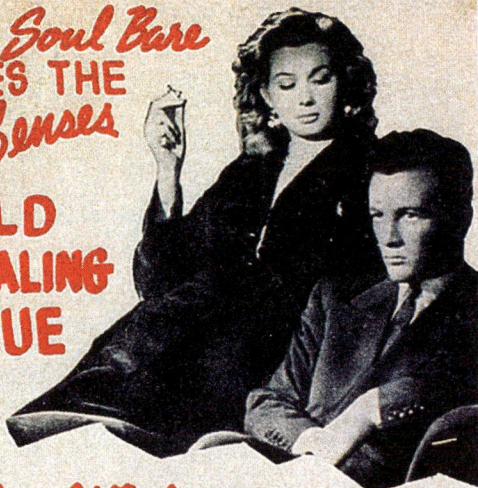

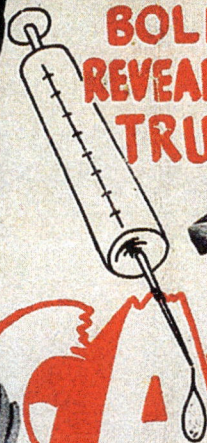

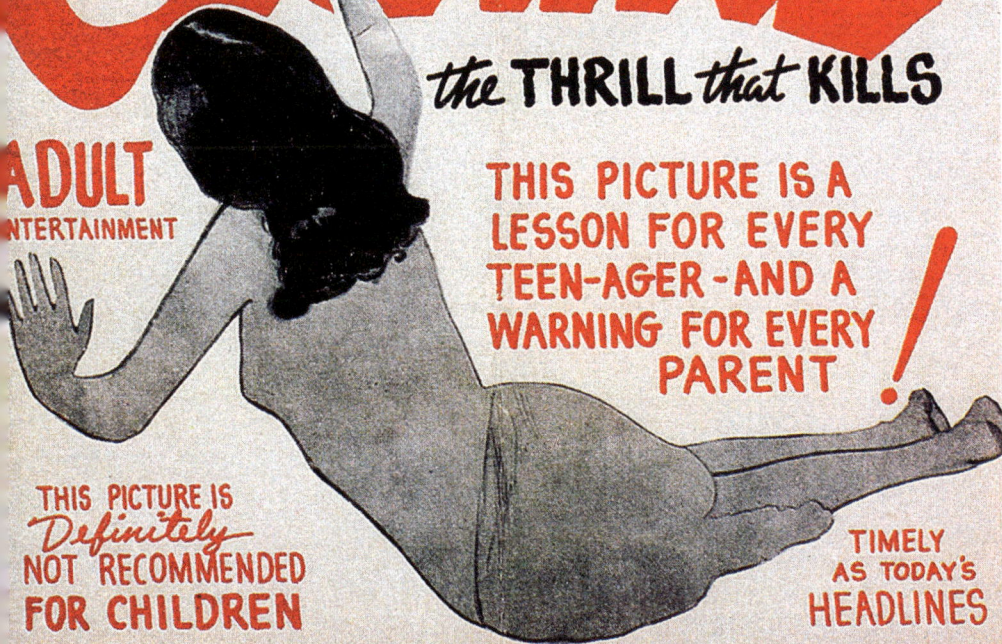

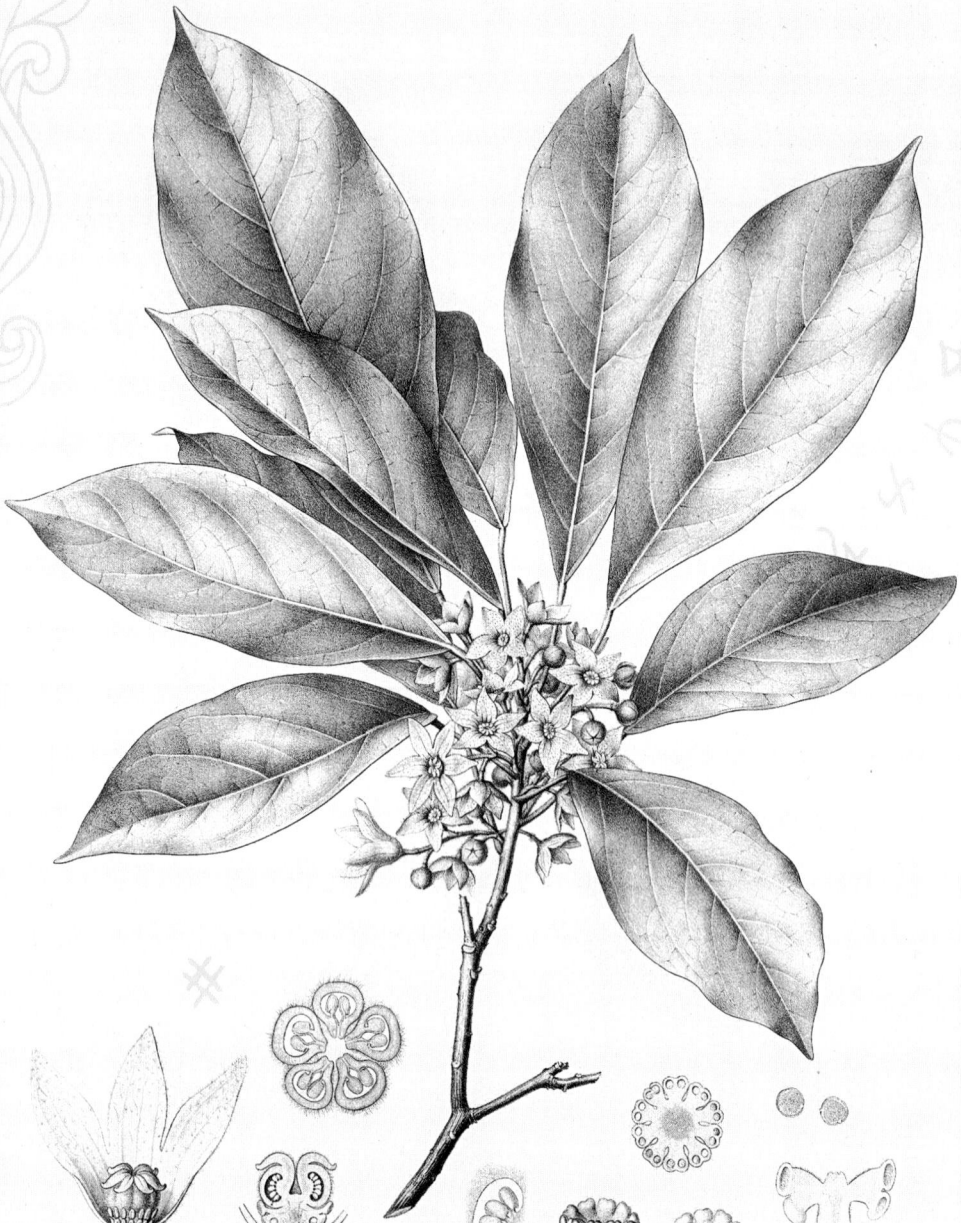

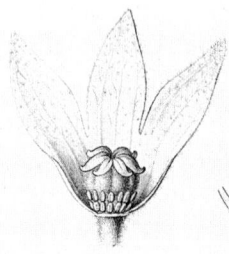

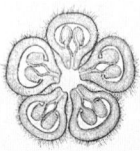

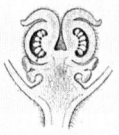

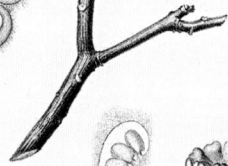

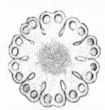

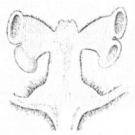

Kola

*Cola acuminata /
Cola nitida*

Kola has been a powerful symbol in West African culture
since at least the eleventh century. Every community has its
own stories, but they all agree on one thing: sharing the nut
represents friendship and respect.

Kola nuts may come from either of two members of the *Cola genus*: *C. acuminata* and *C. nitida*, both evergreen trees of the African rainforests. Their bitter seeds are colourful, irregular, ovoid balls, up to 5cm (2in) long, containing high levels of caffeine, theobromine and other alkaloids. Chewed or brewed as a tea, kola is a stimulant that is considered to restore vitality and curb hunger pangs, and to be addictive. A traditional digestive, tonic, medicine, aphrodisiac, even a dye, it is also, famously, a major ingredient in soft drinks, but West African people will confirm a far higher cultural – and spiritual – importance for the kola nut.

Some Igbo people say Chukwu the creator planted the cola tree for gods and humans alike. Others claim that the gods, who used to bring kola nuts to enjoy with sacrifices left for them by humans, accidently left some behind on Earth. A third tale suggests that Igbo ancestors visited the gods and returned with kola as a parting gift.

Kola is used in ceremonies and, importantly, to honour guests. Decorative *okwa oji* (kola-nut bowls) are still used in Igbo hospitality rituals, while gifts of kola represent gratitude and respect. This is often between or towards chiefs, but the plant's significance resounds throughout society.

To chew kola together implies love and trust. As they age, the seeds split into two irregular halves, which fit exactly into one another. This has come to symbolize courtship and marriage. For the Mamprusi people, chewing the nut with the chief and his court solemnizes and provides witnesses for the union. The nut is also chewed at events such as funerals, naming ceremonies and, crucially, when discussing important matters. Offerings of kola are placed, with prayers, at crossroads or the entrances to anthills, and single nuts sometimes used in divination rituals.

Hans Sloane, the plant collector, botanist and physician, first described kola nuts after seeing seeds from the "Bichy" tree arriving on ships transporting enslaved Akan Africans across the Atlantic. This uncomfortable association did not prevent the exploitation of kola by the West over the following three hundred years.

In spite, or perhaps because of its associations with friendship and trust, kola's bitter taste has occasionally been used to disguise poisons. On receiving a formal gift of kola, therefore, the recipient traditionally hands it back. The donor breaks a little away and tastes it to prove their good intentions.

The Real Thing

Folklore isn't always ancient. It can appear at any time from seemingly nowhere. Sometimes it is manufactured, sometimes it grows, sometimes it is clever marketing, but legends of any kind stick only when they speak to something in us all.

Take Coca-Cola, part of the world's vocabulary for 130-plus years and which has its own set of very strange urban legends, some call "Cokelore". The company is bashful about John Stith Pemberton's original recipe for "coca wine", but it was hardly the only drink on the market in the late nineteenth century with its roots in the new wonder tonic cocaine. Vin Mariani, a French beverage made by mixing Bordeaux wine with coca leaves, was doing a roaring trade, with customers ranging from Popes Leo XIII and Pius X to Jules Verne and Queen Victoria.

The world was genuinely excited about the new drug's possibilities for pain relief. Chloroform and ether had been used for 40 years, but they were blunt instruments. A patient knocked out with chloroform might never return from their induced slumber. Cocaine offered local anaesthesia, either as an injection or rubbed into the afflicted body part. News travelled fast, and not always through medical channels. Sherlock Holmes fans watched the detective dose himself with science's newest marvel and wanted some themselves.

Cocaine reputedly treated sea sickness, toothache, hay fever, even the common cold, via a pocket-sized nasal spray. Tattoo artists injected their clients before wielding other needles; cosmetic surgeons used it to numb in the early days of nose jobs; and if initial proposals that cocaine might be useful in weaning people off morphine and alcohol addiction ultimately turned out to be somewhat wide of the mark, it was not for want of looking for the good the new drug could do.

Pemberton's French Wine Coca, including extract of coca leaves, was launched in 1885, adding kola nut to improve the flavour and add a caffeine kick. The same year, the state of Georgia passed prohibition laws – Pemberton replaced the wine with syrup, carbonated the result as "Coca-Cola" and became the darling of the temperance movement.

Gradually, however, public opinion turned, as cocaine's side effect – addiction – began to show. "Cocaine Monster Throws His Tentacles Around the Nation", screamed the *Los Angeles Herald* on 11 December 1898. The honeymoon was over.

Under new management, Coca-Cola's coca levels had already dropped considerably. As the tide turned on cocaine, any trace elements that Coca-Cola may still have retained (and we will never know; the recipe has always been a closely guarded secret) were removed. Some suggest a tiny amount was retained to justify the name. If so, it had disappeared completely by 1930. Cokelore moved on, too, to Santa Claus and tooth dissolving. The conspiracy theorists will always be with us.

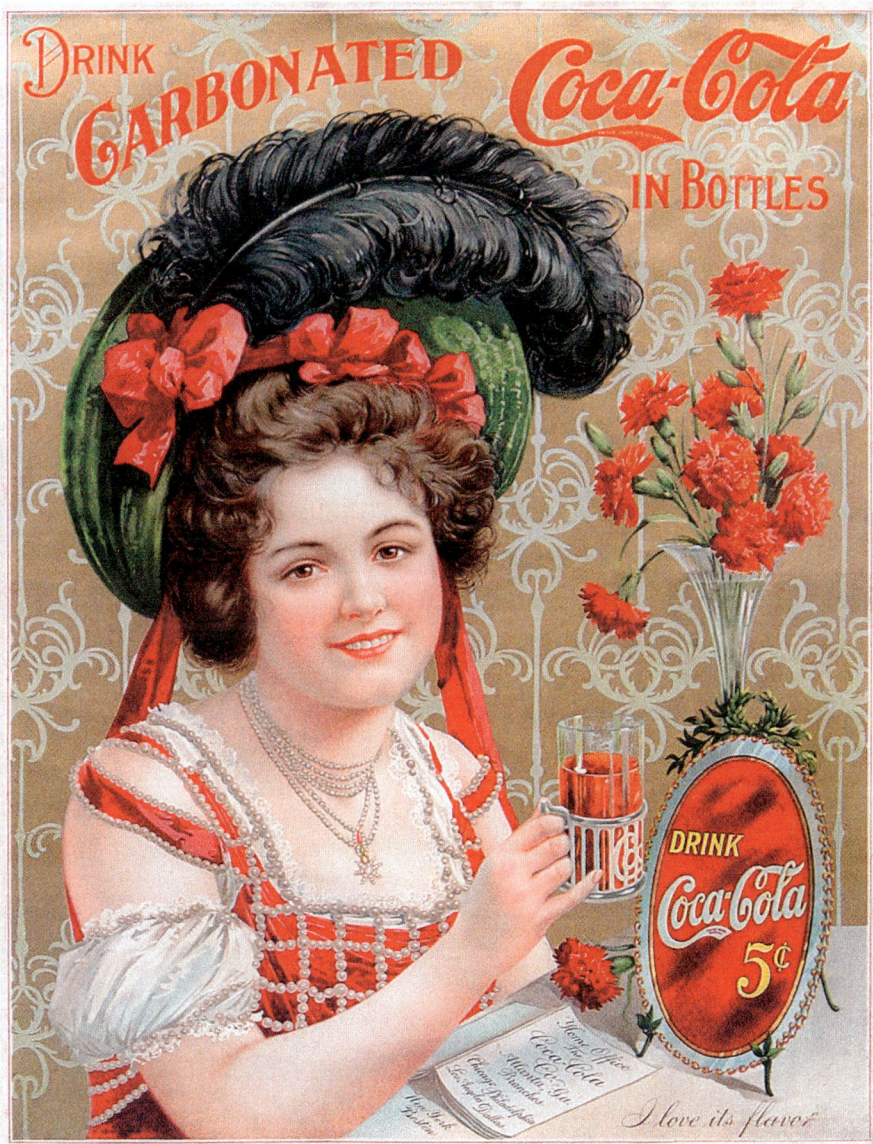

Above A 1902 Coca-Cola advertisement featuring
Hilda Clark. At the time, Coca-Cola contained
cocaine as well as caffeine.

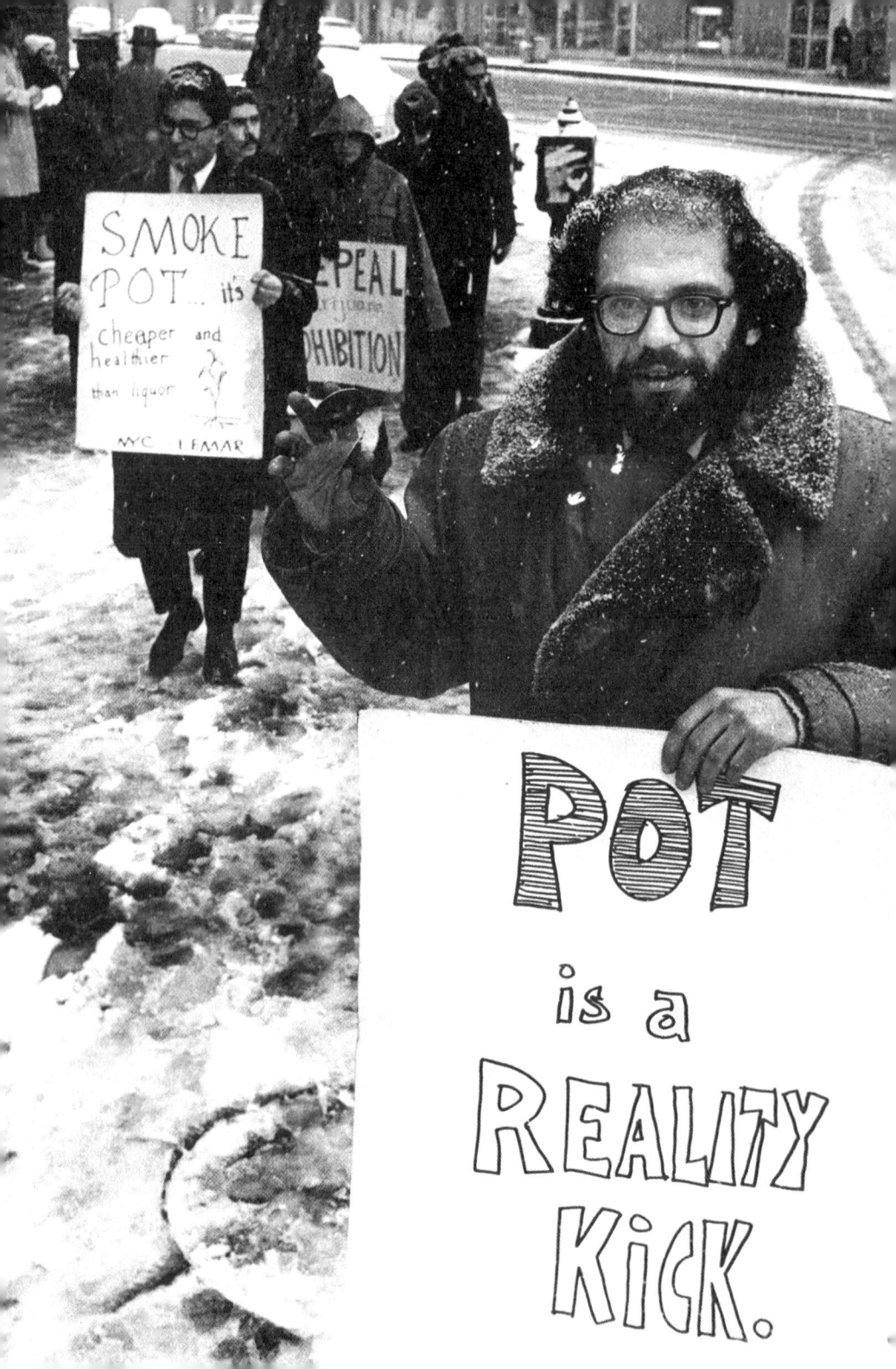

Hop Heads, Jive Talk and the Beat Generation

A famous scene in the 1957 Hollywood musical *Funny Face* sees Fred Astaire and Kay Thompson in black polo necks, beard for him, beret for her, sneaking into a Parisian cellar bar trying to pass themselves off as the new youth bugaboo: beatniks.

Of course, the name itself hadn't yet been coined. That would come the following year, in an article by *San Francisco Chronicle* columnist Herb Caen, combining the word beat with another threat to all-American values, the Soviet *sputnik*, but the damage was done. Mainstream movies were making fun of the beat generation, and the beat generation didn't like it.

The classic stereotype – head-to-toe black, goatees, glasses and Gauloises – is still a popular fancy dress option, and it still raises a slight smirk. While it also includes copious use of bongos, however, the word *beat* does not refer to music. First used by author Jack Kerouac in 1948, it was intended to convey the weariness of a youth "beat" by the generation before it – beat by war, conventionality and conformity.

Squinting through smoke-wreathed darkness in New York's Greenwich Village, existentialist Parisian cellar clubs and the radical bookstores of San Francisco, earnest young people discussed ideas and listened to Charlie Parker, Miles Davis and the chanson française of Juliette Gréco through a haze of substances. Alcohol was universal, as was marijuana. Morphine and the trade-named amphetamine Benzedrine were also common, but this would also be the first generation to experiment with psychedelics, including peyote, psilocybin, ayahuasca and, later, the synthetic LSD. More tragically, heroin was also popular, especially among jazz musicians. Substance abuse would claim the lives of far too many, including Charlie Parker (aged 34), John Coltrane (aged 40) and Billie Holliday (aged 44).

While the beat generation took its ideas very seriously, it was less straight-faced about itself. "Jive talk" was a constantly evolving, dark-humoured argot garnered from pulp novels, film noir, street slang and bebop improvisation. Jazz poet/musician Babs Gonzales tried to pickle it in his *Boptionary*, but he was clutching at eels. Max Décharné's later lexicon, *Straight from the Fridge, Dad* (2000), is probably as close as we'll get. The sheer number of words for the drug scene is extraordinary. Hep cats might start the evening with a little A-bomb juice, tonsil paint or neck oil (liquor) until they were "screwed, blued and tattooed", before joining the weed hounds and grasshoppers already "going steady with Mary Jane" (marijuana) in partaking of a little righteous bush in the form of roaches, jive sticks or (with apologies to *Harry Potter* fans) muggles. Snowbirds might take a ski-ride on some nose candy (cocaine) while hardened opium fans kicked the gong around.

It's no wonder poor Fred Astaire was out of his depth.

Opposite Allen Ginsberg leads a group of protestors advocating for the use of marijuana in 1965.

Chapter 7:
Freaky Fungi

The idea of "magic mushrooms"
is so well known it is almost
a cliché, but perhaps the
freakiest thing about "freaky
fungi" is how little we know
about them. Assumed to be
some kind of weird "plants"
for millennia, it was only
comparatively recently that
fungus was allotted its own
kingdom: neither plant nor
animal but "something else".

Mycology, the study of fungi, has always been the Cinderella of science. The discipline limped along piecemeal for centuries, often conducted by amateur scientists laughed at as cranks in their day.

erious work on the kingdom of fungi has only come into its own in more recent decades. Many of the estimated 2,500,000 species remain undescribed; many more, perhaps, undiscovered. Yet even within the species we know so far may be found some of the most psychoactive substances on earth.

Nearly everything we know about the various hallucinogenic and otherwise mind-altering effects of certain mushrooms may be attributed to the work of indigenous peoples across the world who discovered, presumably the hard way, what they could do. They learned where to look, what to look for, which species were good to eat, which could kill you and which could, in the hands of a skilled practitioner, take you "somewhere else".

Like psychoactive plants, each mushroom genus/species works on the mind in different ways. Fly agaric (*Amanita muscaria*), for example, has an entirely different constitution to ergot (*Claviceps purpurea*). Even the "psilocybin" group of fungi, which contain various psychoactive ingredients, the most widely known being psilocybin, is more an informal group of loosely related fungi than a specific genus. They range from the notorious laughing mushrooms (*Gymnopilus junonius*), that allegedly saw ninth-century Buddhist nuns dancing through Japanese forests, to the classic magic mushrooms of South America (*Psilocybe*) though even these can vary in composition. While it is becoming clearer

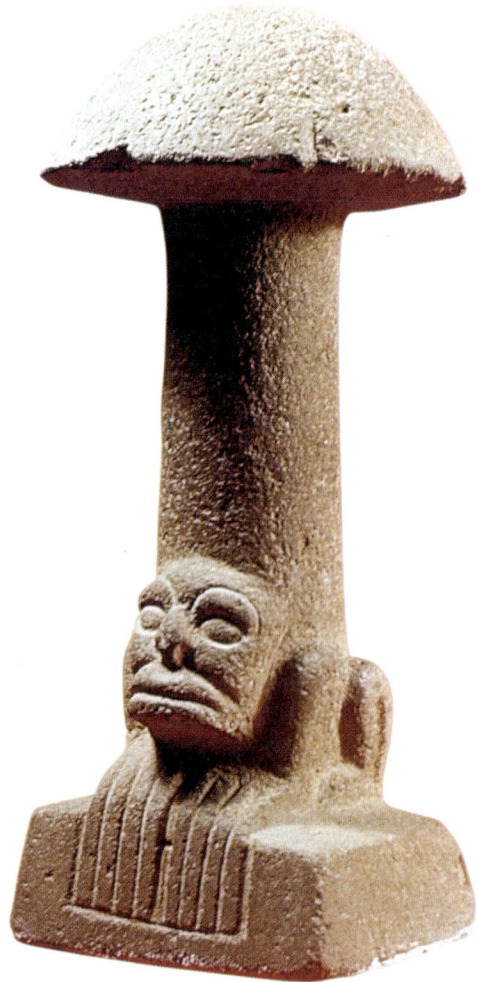

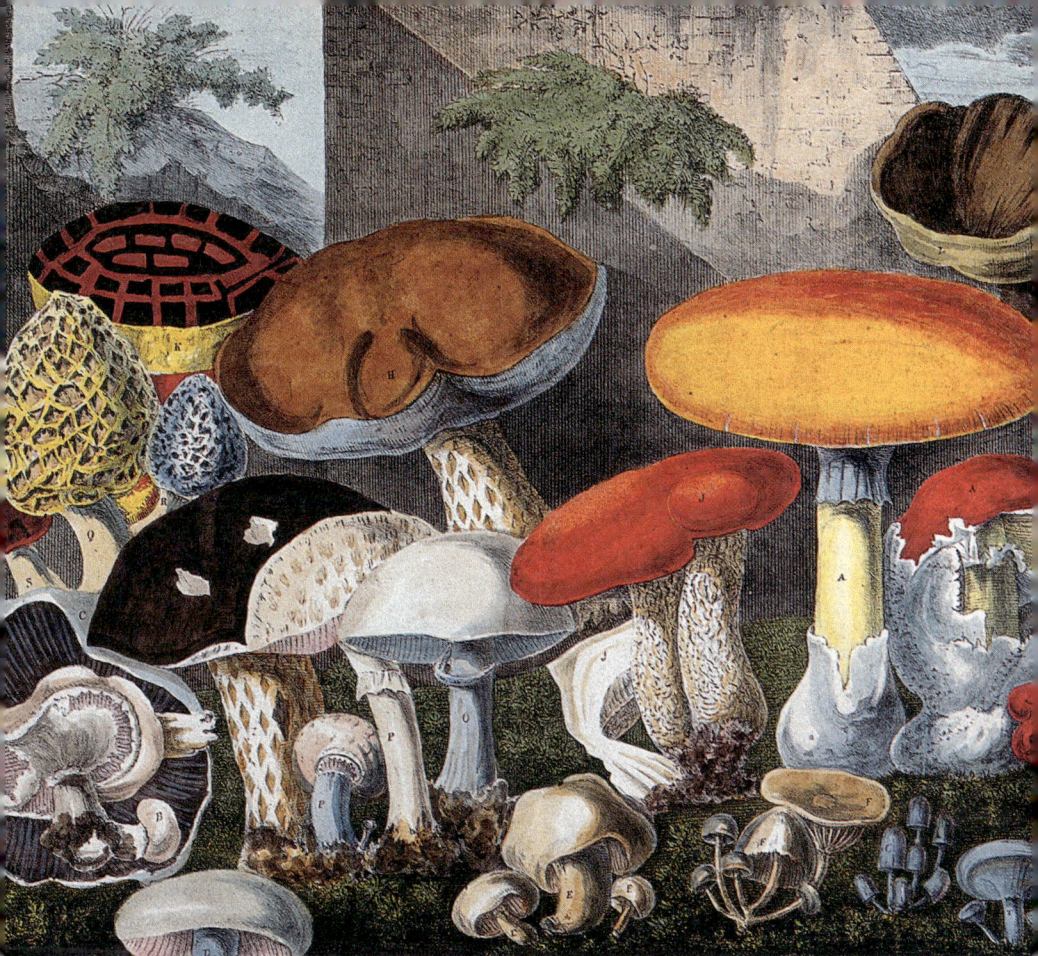

how certain psychoactive substances work – we now know, for example, that psilocybin is converted by the body to the hallucinogenic substance psilocin – we do not know exactly how the various combinations of less common compounds also found within individual species work on the human body. This is both terrifying and exciting. They could kill or seriously damage us or be the gateway to a medical breakthrough.

We are used to Western science being the culmination of centuries' worth of previous, mainly lab-based, work. For mycologists, Planet Earth is still the Wild West. Grateful for any new insights into the way this strange kingdom works, "ethnomycologists" look for other more tangible clues, within the social and cultural practices of the indigenous people who already understand and, more importantly, respect the fungi they work with.

Opposite A Mayan stone sculpure in the shape of a mushroom with an animal on the bottom, from Guatemala.

Above An illustration of 19 species of edible fungi, including horse and field mushrooms.

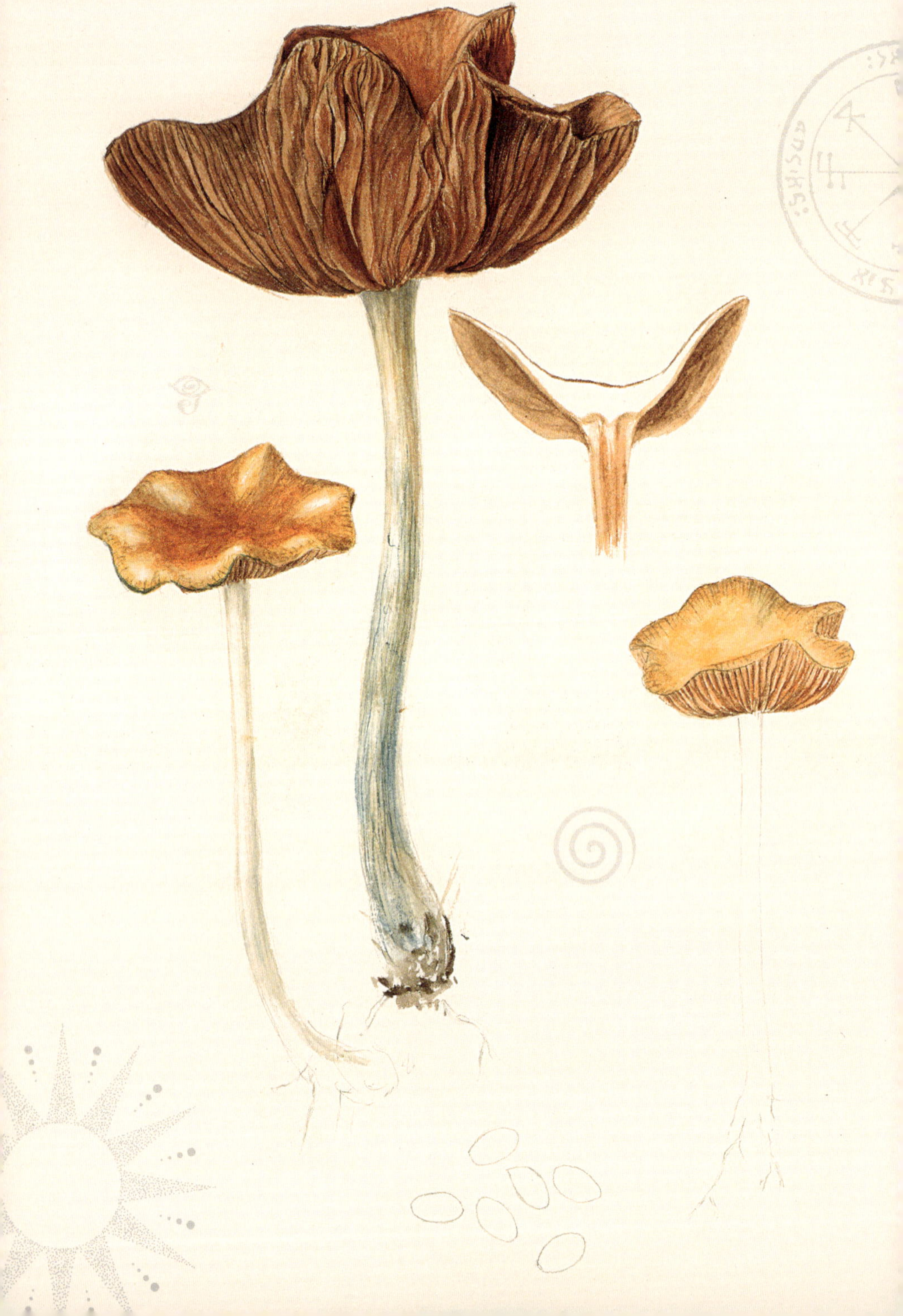

Magic mushrooms: *Psilocybe*

Deep in the curious, lunar-like landscape of Tassili n'Ajjer,
Algeria, lie caves filled with paintings dating back to
c. 6000 BCE.

Some of the figures are running, others carry mushrooms with dotted lines linking the fungi to their heads. It is unlikely these can be conclusively proved to be magic mushrooms, but psilocybin is hardly rare; it occurs in around 180 identified species, lending the *Psilocybe* genus its scientific name.

Psilocybin is a *prodrug*, converted inside the body to the psychoactive compound psilocin. It acts on all the senses, creating auditory and visual hallucinations, as well as affecting emotion, cognition and concepts of time. A user's sense of memory may be enhanced, but they can also experience trauma and/or depression. Experienced shamans use such sensations to diagnose illness and seek advice during ritual consumption.

Archaeological sites across Central America, especially in Guatemala, have yielded around two hundred curious "mushroom stones". These strange, squat little people, animals and spirits, are usually but not always seated, wearing enormous mushroom headdresses, which suggests some kind of ancient fungus cult. Dating them is difficult – estimates have placed them anywhere from 2000 BCE to the early years of the first century CE – but they are often associated with the Mayan civilization.

For the Aztecs, *Psilocybe* mushrooms were *Teonanácatl* (divine flesh), considered "flowers"

and used in rituals, to the horror of their conquerors, the Spanish, who did their best to obliterate such heresy. Outraged Roman Catholic missionaries described poor natives tempted by the Devil to horrific cruelties and crazed madness, claiming visions of demons and snakes. These accounts make distasteful reading today but provide a window into how people used mushrooms before they were bludgeoned into Christian conformity. We learn, for example, how the menfolk ventured into the hills by night to pray, waiting for a certain breeze to blow at dawn, the optimum time to gather the sacred mushrooms.

Perhaps understandably, mushroom use disappeared underground, so deeply that in 1916 an American botanist even suggested that the sacred mushrooms and peyote cactus must be the same thing and that cunning natives, who could never be trusted, kept pointing out harmless fungi to distract the authorities. In the 1930s things began to change, especially when Richard Evans Schultes, the father of ethnobotany, visited the Mazatec people of Mexico in a spirit of learning rather than domination. In 1957, Robert Gordon Wasson wrote his seminal article "Seeking the Magic Mushroom" for *Life* magazine and the secret was blown wide open.

When Gordon Met Maria

Middle-class, upstanding and a respectable United States
citizen, as well as a vice president of J.P. Morgan, Robert
Gordon Wasson shocked America when he became the first
known non-indigenous man to take psychedelic fungi, in 1957.

T he two women also involved in the story behind *Life* magazine's "Seeking the Magic Mushroom" were quietly sidelined. The story of magic mushrooms is essentially one of corruption, exploitation and, frankly, misogyny, and while Wasson was not directly responsible for any of the above (indeed, he would be horrified at the later outcomes), that magazine article opened the door to excess.

Wasson had been brought up, like most Americans, to be deeply suspicious of fungi. His Russian-born wife Valentina Pavlovna Guerken was the exact opposite, and together the couple came up with the concepts of *mycophilic* and *mycophobic* for cultures that, respectively, love and fear fungi. In 1956, the couple went on an (funded, unknown to them, by the CIA) expedition to Oaxaca, Mexico, to seek counsel from the indigenous Mazatec healer María Sabina Magdalena García.

Sabina came from a line of village healers and participated in her first velada (sacred mushroom ceremony) at the age of seven. Paralyzed by grief at the death of her first husband, she turned to her *los Niños Santos* (Holy Children – magic mushrooms) and discovered a gift for healing.

Sabina was initially reluctant to reveal her secrets but eventually relented and Wasson's tiny group took part in a velada. "Seeking the Magic Mushroom" was

respectful of Sabina's work, but Wasson's publishers – and America as a whole – sensationalized it. Valentina's article "I Ate the Sacred Mushrooms", appeared in *This Week* magazine just one week later, but the very idea of a respectable housewife doing exactly the same thing as her spouse was too much for 1950s America. Valentina would die the following year and, until recently, society seems very happy to have buried her name behind that of her husband.

There would be even worse backlash for María Sabina. The publicity opened the way for a destructive hippy-trail of foreigners besieging the villages, wanting to get stoned. The Mazatec community blamed her for defiling the velada; the Global North accused her of drug peddling. Her house was burned down, and she was constantly harassed. Perhaps worst of all, she believed that exploitation by the outside world lost her the power to heal via her "children". She died in poverty in 1985, famous, notorious and sad.

Opposite The front cover of *This Week* showing the sensationalised feature "I Ate the Sacred Mushrooms".

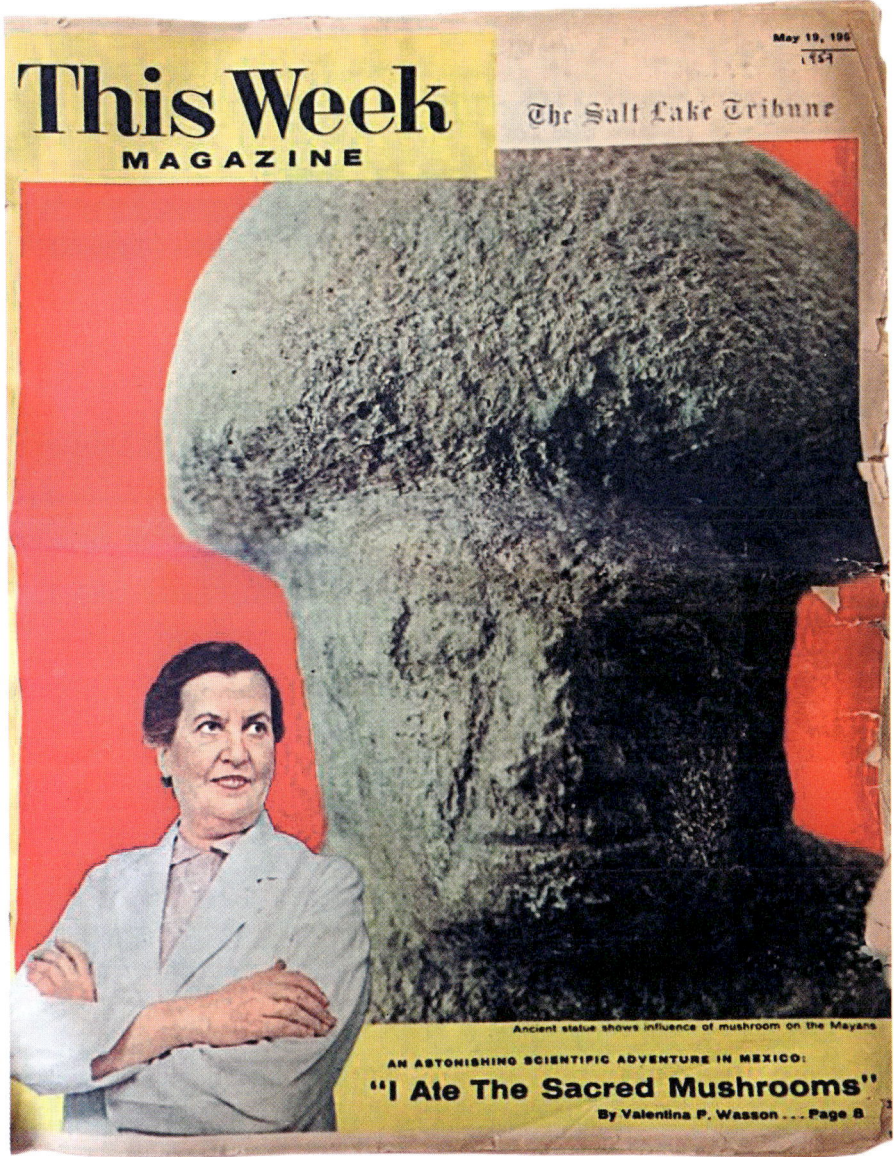

May 19, 196

This Week
MAGAZINE

The Salt Lake Tribune

Ancient statue shows influence of mushroom on the Mayans

AN ASTONISHING SCIENTIFIC ADVENTURE IN MEXICO:

"I Ate The Sacred Mushrooms"

By Valentina P. Wasson . . . Page 8

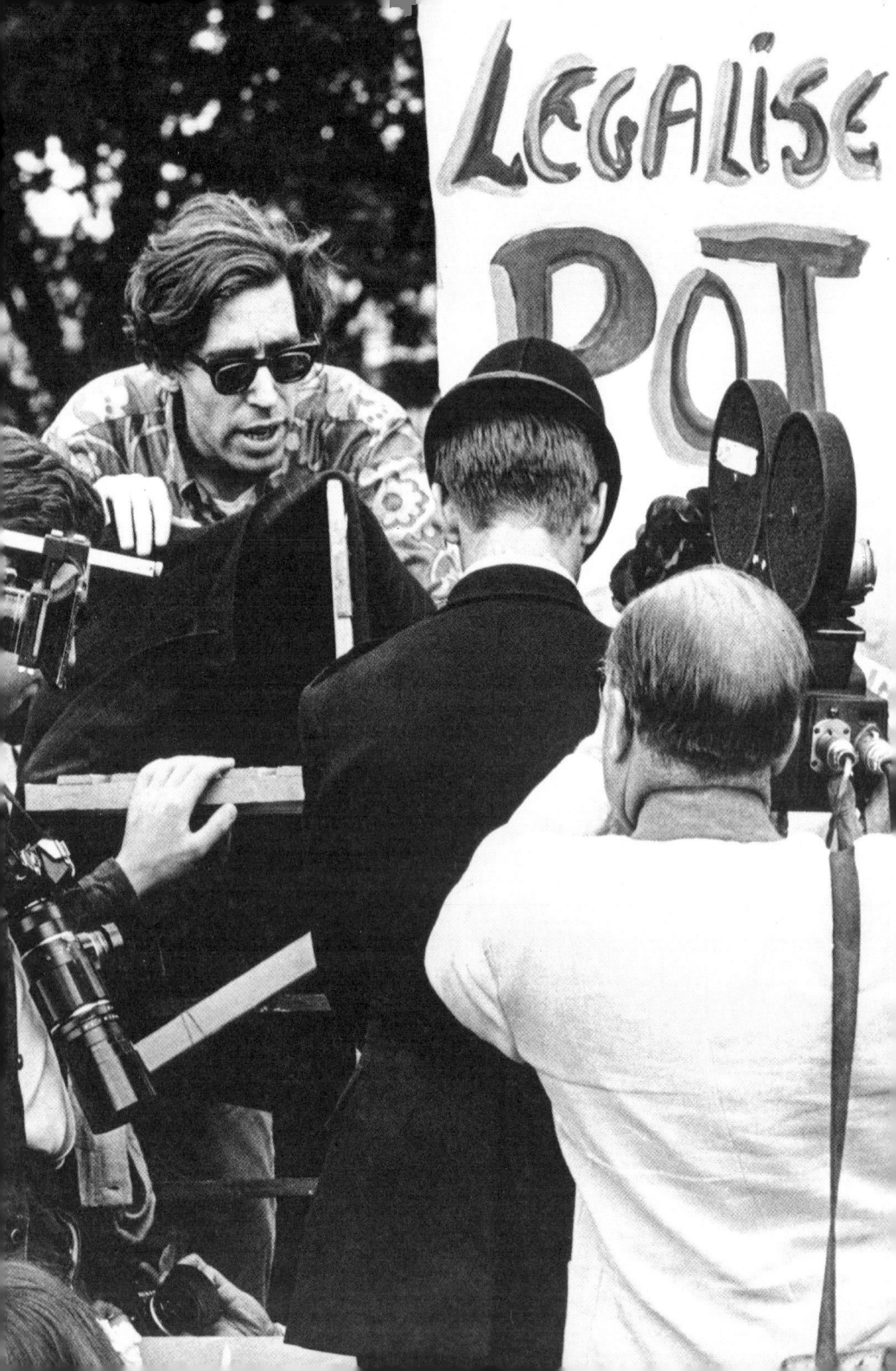

Turn on, Tune in, Drop Out:
Counterculture v. the CIA

As a young lecturer in the psychology department of Harvard University, Timothy Leary tasted psilocybin mushrooms for the first time in 1960. The experience would change his life.

Leary became convinced that the road to higher consciousness was to be discovered through the use of psychedelics and, with colleague Richard Alpert (aka Ram Dass), proposed a radical new research programme. Over three, heady years, the Harvard Psilocybin Project undertook a series of mind-blowing studies, at first on a self-selecting group of volunteers including graduate students and the researchers themselves.

The Concord Prison Experiment saw Leary's team administering psilocybin to 32 maximum security prison inmates to see if their experiences might reduce repeat offending. The team also ingested the compound, ostensibly to create a sense of shared equality, but with the side effect that everyone was under the influence of entheogenic hallucinogens throughout the experiment.

It was the 1960s.

The project's other major study was the Marsh Chapel Experiment conducted by graduate student Walter N. Pahnke, under the supervision of Leary and Alpert, on Good Friday, 1962, where divinity student

Opposite Police prevent people advocating for legalsing marijuana from entering Hyde Park. While people were allowed to express their views for legalising the substance, they were not allowed to bring signs.

volunteers from a seminary school went down into the chapel's basement to listen to the Easter service being held upstairs. Half had taken psilocybin, the others a placebo. Every student that had taken the mushrooms had strange, "religious" experiences; the rest watched in puzzlement.

Both studies were pronounced a success at the time, although much discussion – both negative and positive – has arisen since, but Harvard was not happy. Leary and Alpert were accused of safety transgressions, flawed analysis and ethical breaches, including pressurizing students into taking part and giving psilocybin to undergraduates off-campus. The project was closed down and both academics were dismissed.

Leary was undeterred. Working with beat poet Allen Ginsberg, he popularized psychedelics among artists, authors, musicians and intellectuals as 1960s counterculture gradually enveloped America.

Lysergic acid diethylamide, better known by its initials LSD, had been synthesized in 1938, by chemist Albert Hofmann who was looking for a safe way to use medicinally the naturally occurring alkaloid in ergot (see p. 127). The new compound was marketed by the Swiss laboratory Sandoz as a psychiatric cure-all and many, including Timothy Leary and Richard Alpert, were very interested indeed in finding out exactly what it could do.

Perhaps surprisingly, however, LSD was actually (and covertly) brought to the USA by the CIA, as part of an exhaustive search for drugs that could be used in brainwashing and torture during intelligence gathering.

Project MKUltra was founded in 1953, at the height of the Cold War, with the aim of finding the ultimate "truth drug". In charge was the chemist and spymaster Sidney Gottlieb, later dubbed Poisoner-in-Chief, who arranged in secret to purchase Sandoz's entire supply of LSD for $240,000. This was administered in various dosages to prisoners, mental health patients, heroin addicts and prostitutes; citizens who had little or no idea they were part of an ongoing experiment. In one, not unique, example, agents from Operation Midnight Climax administered LSD to men visiting CIA-created brothels and observed them via two-way mirrors, while the prostitutes were directed to question them to see if the men would reveal secrets, or were suggestible. The agents running the projects assumed that the men would be too embarrassed to admit to anything later.

Project MKUltra, along with an alarming number of other unsavoury undercover practices, would be unmasked during the 1975 Rockefeller Commission, but this was long after LSD had escaped its CIA clutches and been discovered by an altogether happier 1960s counterculture. As various cultural figures, from Aldous Huxley to the Beatles, embraced the new substance, LSD was denounced as a threat to American values, even potentially perilous to the nation's efforts in the Vietnam War. By 1968 it was a Schedule 1 controlled substance.

Leary continued to lobby for the drug, and when asked whether he thought it dangerous, famously replied that a motor car was dangerous if used improperly. A master of the catchphrase, Timothy Leary introduced the idea of "set and setting" (the mindset with which someone enters the process of taking psychedelics and the setting in which it takes place) and uttered one of the most famous quotations of the hippy era: "turn on, tune in, drop out", which appeared on a spoken word album of the same name in 1966.

The ultimate anti-establishment figure, Leary was arrested 36 times, perhaps for following the spirit of another famous decree: "Think for yourself and question authority."

In later years, Leary switched his attention to computers, particularly entranced by the concept of virtual reality. Entreating his followers to "turn on, boot up, jack in", he declared the PC to be "the LSD of the 1990s". History will decide if he was right, but it is, perhaps, no coincidence that some of Silicon Valley's great entrepreneurs, including Steve Jobs and Elon Musk, have been exponents of synthesized psychedelic substances.

Opposite Timothy Leary mediating at the Village Gate Theatre in 1960.

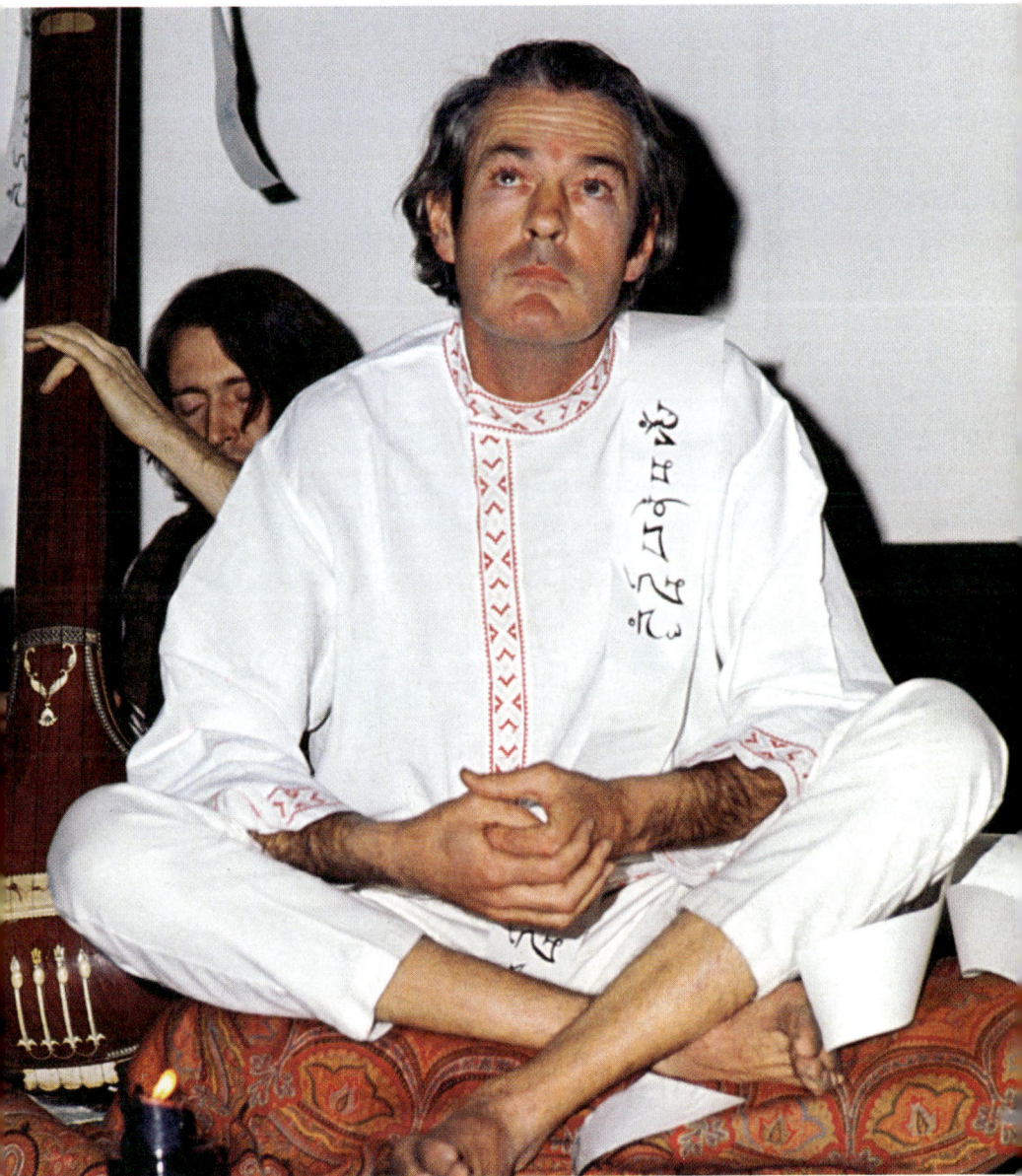

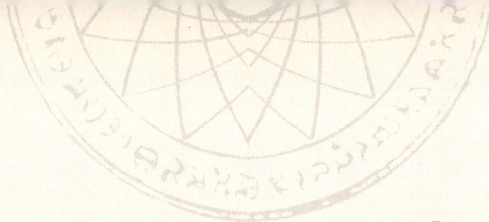

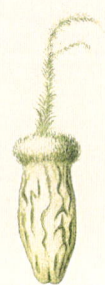

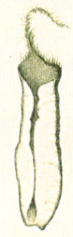

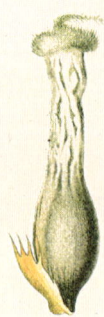

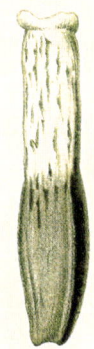

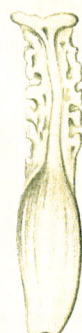

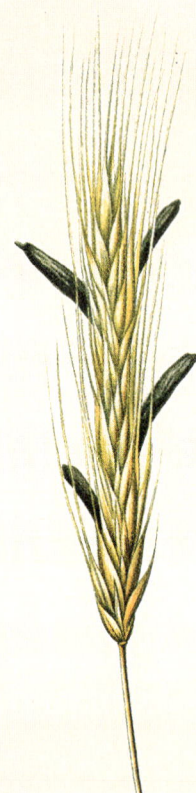

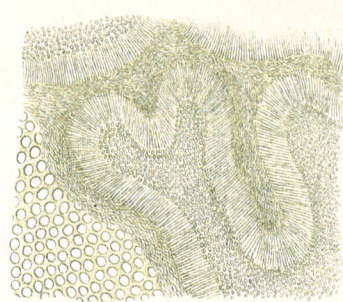

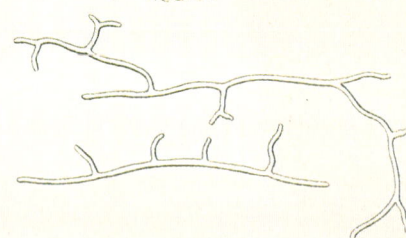

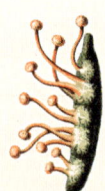

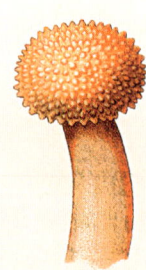

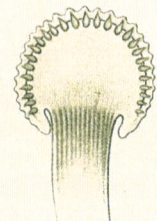

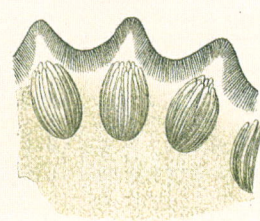

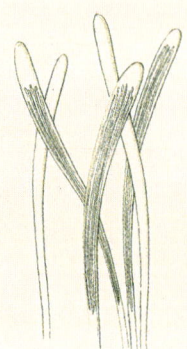

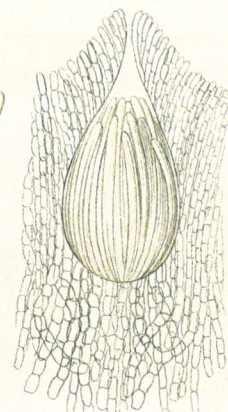

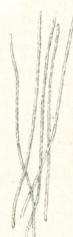

Ergot

Claviceps purpurea

We may never know what went on during the Eleusinian
Mysteries of ancient Greece, but from descriptions of the
festival's frenzied rites, some scholars have been reminded of
the effects of a fungal parasite, *Claviceps*.

*E*rgot is French for a cock's spur, and the tiny black sclerotia (fruiting bodies) of *Claviceps* which grow on grasses, especially rye (*Secale cereale*), in damp years, are well nicknamed. The dangers of ergot were first noticed by the ancient Assyrians, and the Greeks did not usually eat infected grain. If ergot was indeed used in the Eleusinian Mysteries, partakers would have actively invited the fungus's strange convulsions and hallucinations.

Rye did not appear further north in Europe until the coming of Christianity, so earlier wisdom was lost. Several instances of "diabolical possession" have since been potentially attributed to ergot poisoning.

"St Anthony's Fire", named for an obscure hermit-saint, manifested in two ways: convulsions, delirium and hallucinations, or a creeping gangrene, which caused sufferers to lose fingers, toes, ears and even noses. Victims also experienced a burning "holy fire" as their blood vessels contracted. The first hospital of the Order of St Anthony was founded in 1095, and proved successful in treating ergotism, though this may have had less to do with prayers than being built in a region unaffected by the fungus.

Although the cause of ergotism was tracked down to infected rye in 1676, the problem persisted (and still persists in very small part) because it was not easy to entirely clean the grain. Popular fear of disease manfested in *feldgeister* (field spirits) such as the German Kornmutter (grain mother), a figure who lived in the ears of corn, and whose children were tiny ergot spurs. She was known under many names across Eastern Europe, including the *Roggenmuhme* (rye aunt) who lured children into her field and sent them insane as she suckled them from iron teats. The *Roggenwolf* also abducted children and has been associated with the madness of werewolves.

As so often with toxins, ergot had its admirers. The muscle spasms suffered by victims sometimes caused pregnant women to miscarry, so it became a (dangerous) backstreet abortifacient. Research has led to another use: ergot alkaloids from this fungus became the inspiration to develop synthetic drugs to alleviate Parkinson's disease symptoms.

There is one direct result of ergot specific to this book. On 19 April 1943, chemist Albert Hofmann was attempting to synthesize *Claviceps*'s alkaloids for potential pharmaceutical use when he accidentally absorbed some into his skin. After a brighter cycle ride home than usual, an event now celebrated annually as Bicycle Day, he realized he had invented LSD.

The Summer of Love

The date is 1967, the place San Francisco, the people young. Around 100,000 of them are travelling across the United States wearing flowers in their hair, ready for the party of their lives.

The idea of an "alternative" culture had been seeping into comfortable, conservative, post-war America since 1945, at first through the beat writers and musicians of the 1950s nibbling at the unprotected heel of an affluent but brittle society. On the surface America exhaled confidence – they were going to put a man on the moon, for heaven's sake – but a growing faction of middle-class baby boomers was disillusioned. Seeing the materialism of a society prepared to engage in nuclear war or send them to die in Vietnam, they were beginning to want out.

Hippies (from the term *hip*, used to describe the previous, 1950s beat generation) embraced an alternative lifestyle, wearing colourful clothing, growing their hair and taking full advantage of the new contraceptive pill. While some suggested such "flower children" dropped out because they could afford to – leaving, for example, Black Americans to fight for even basic rights – many sincerely believed in their bohemian lifestyle based around peace, love and an ultimate quest to find spiritual awakening.

Such fulfilment was, for many, to be achieved through the use of psychedelic stimulants such as psilocybin mushrooms and LSD, the synthetic drug based around naturally occurring ergot alkaloids.

The movement's epicentre was in San Francisco's run-down Haight-Ashbury district, beloved for its cheap property and concentration of musicians, writers and artists. The Merry Pranksters, followers of Ken Kesey (of *One Flew over the Cuckoo's Nest* fame), promoted the psychedelic lifestyle through "happenings"; others, including the San Francisco Mime Troupe, took a more political approach. From Lawrence Ferlinghetti's City Lights bookstore, beloved of beat poets since 1953, to America's first great headshop, the Psychedelic Shop, which opened in 1966 as a safe way of buying hallucinogenic substances, the district had everything a bohemian could want.

All eventually converged in 1967 at Golden Gate Park for a substance-fuelled musical love-in later dubbed the Summer of Love. Bands including Jefferson Airplane, the Grateful Dead and the Byrds joined artists such as Janis Joplin and Jimi Hendrix, psychedelics were taken, love was spread and so was the concept – to New York, California, Denver, even to a Great British stately home, Woburn Abbey.

It was all getting … intense. On 6 October, a mock funeral for "the death of the hippie" was held in Buena Vista Park, San Francisco. It proved premature. The off-Broadway musical *Hair* opened 11 days later. It had been only a few months, but the world would never be the same again.

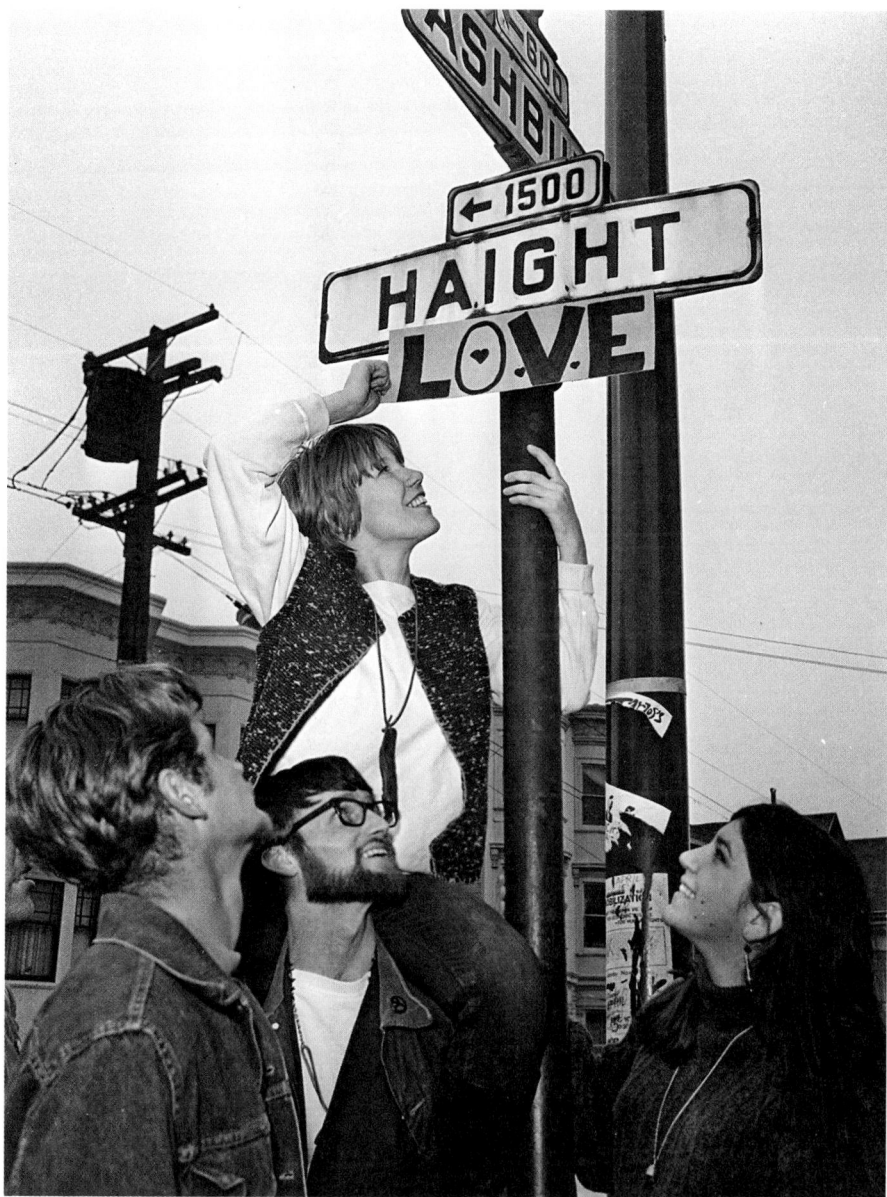

Above No room for hate: The sign for
Haight Street is changed to 'Love' in 1967.

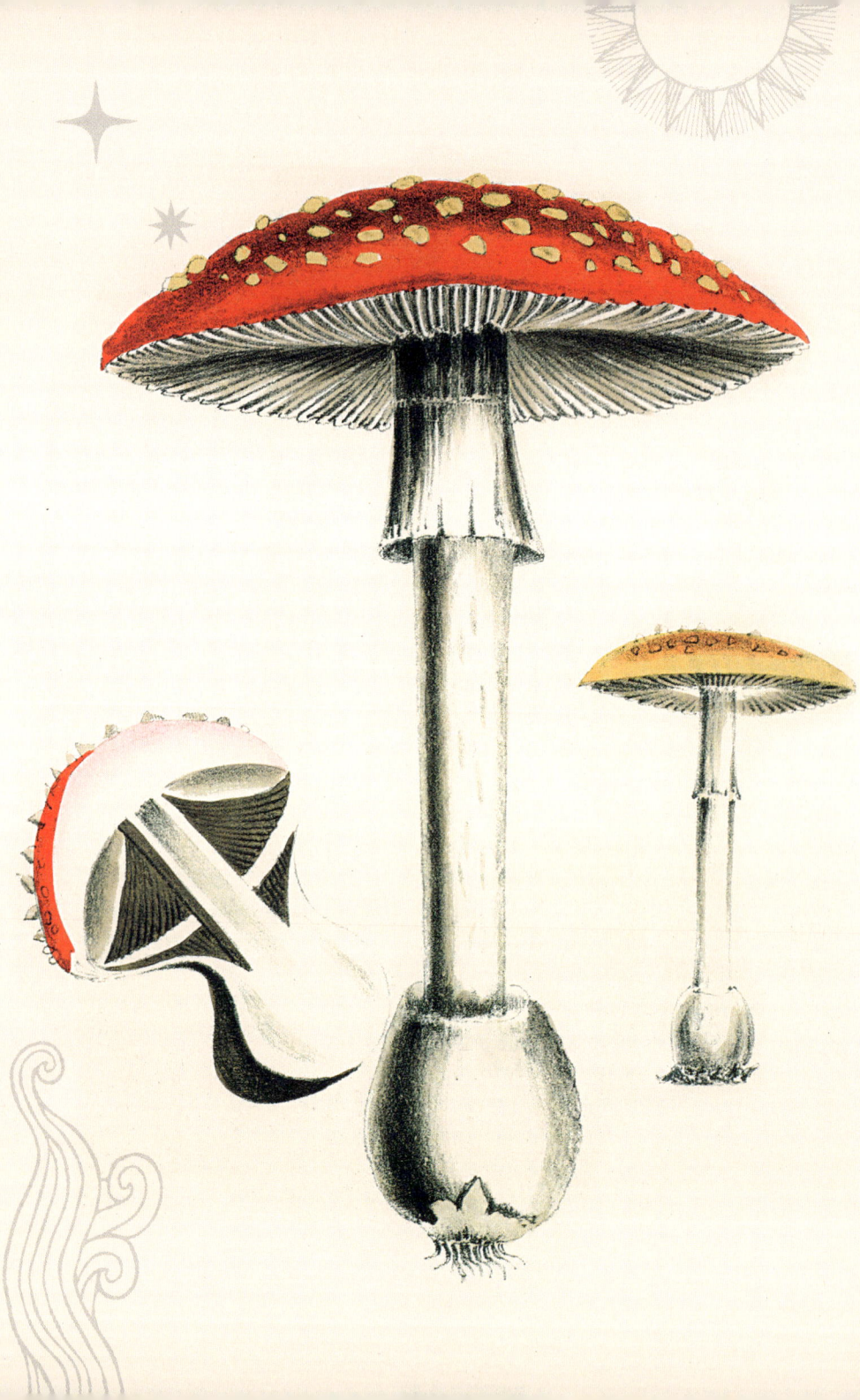

Fly agaric

Amanita muscaria

Big Raven needed to return a lost whale to the sea. Vahiyinin, the sky god, spat on the ground and told Big Raven to eat the little mushrooms with spotted red hats that sprang up there.

Big Raven did so and grew strong enough to carry the whale through the air to the ocean. The Koryak people of Siberia continue the story, revealing that Big Raven then asked if the little spirits could grow permanently on earth.

The classic fairytale toadstool, *Amanita muscaria* is the most recognizable member of the fungus kingdom. It carries a heavy cultural burden. The subject of "cute" art and Christmas ornaments, it also has a darker folklore that ranges from its associations with fairies and witches to theories about it enabling Santa Claus's reindeer to fly. At least part of this confused heritage may be traced to a few basic truths. Fly agaric is a hallucinogen. People who consumed it *did* imagine they could fly, and reindeer really do seek out *Amanita*'s fruiting bodies, though it is unlikely any creature ever pulled an airborne sleigh.

Amanita is a large fungal genus that includes both deadly and edible species. A small amount of the ibotenic acid in *A. muscaria* (and its cousin the panther cap, *A. pantherina*) converts to the deliriant muscimol inside the human body. Shamans use the realistic, colourful hallucinations, sense of detachment and illusions of energy and strength derived from the fungus as a mediator between worlds, to commune with ancestors, diagnose illness and seek advice, but it is a strange beast. Nausea, convulsions, sweating and blurred vision may accompany the other effects, plus fits of either terror or ecstasy before sudden sleep. Or it may keep you awake. *Amanita* is unpredictable. In some communities only the shaman ingested it first hand. The rest of the ibotenic acid, along with some of the converted muscimol, passed through their bodies, leading to the notorious practice of ritualized urine drinking.

In modern Europe, news of strange peoples who herded reindeer, ate mystical toadstools and underwent ceremonies of crazed raving followed by sudden lethargy were largely dismissed as travellers' tales. In 1730, however, Philipp Johann von Strahlenberg, a Swedish officer captured by the Russians, published an account of the 12 years he spent as a prisoner of war, living among the Koryak, in a magical land of ice, hot springs, volcanos and shamanistic ritual, including his observations on the ritual use of fly agaric.

Chacruna

Psychotria viridis

As the daughter of the sky god gave birth, she broke her finger,
and from it grew the woody caapi vine liana. Her sister also
broke a finger, which became the chacruna tree.

Or perhaps chacruna and its spiritual "sister", caapi (see p. 135) are two of the seven plants that burst from the body of the great rainbow-hued boa Shiu Amarun, who, say the Quechua people, was slain by Atacapi, the many-headed serpent of chaos. Maybe they sprouted from the grave of Manco Cápac, the semi-legendary founder of the Inca civilization. Whichever story is told about the two major ingredients in ayahuasca, they always appear together. Even the name "chacruna" comes from the Quechua word *chaqruy*, "to mix", because neither plant is good without the other.

Psychotria viridis is a skinny shrub from the coffee family which grows to around 5m (16ft) in height and whose leaves contain a remarkable amount of naturally occurring *N*-dimethyltryptamine. Better known to the world as DMT, this is the substance that gives ayahuasca its hallucinatory kick, but on its own chacruna is nothing special. An enzyme called monoamine oxidase (MAO) in the body neutralizes the DMT before it can reach the brain.

Banisteriopsis caapi, however, contains harmala alkaloids which inhibit the MAO enzyme. This action may not only reduce the breakdown of the body's own chemical messengers, including serotonin, but can help reduce the breakdown of DMT, resulting in a state of euphoria. On its own you need large amounts of caapi to get much of a kick. Put the two together and those chemical messengers can tell the brain a whole other story, resulting in hallucinogenic fireworks, but also in unpleasant side effects – including vomiting, nausea, breathing difficulties, chest pains and fainting.

DMT is illegal in many countries of the world. Not so those of the Amazon basin. Peru's National Institute of Culture has even declared the traditional uses of ayahuasca to be a practice of National Cultural Heritage.

In the United States the brew has followed in the footsteps of the Native American Church (see p. 183) and found sanctuary within the 1993 Religious Freedom Restoration Act. Two churches, with the spiritual use of ayahuasca at their core, are exempt from federal ban. Santo Daime, founded in the 1930s, combines aspects of several religions including folk Catholicism, African animism and South American shamanism. União do Vegetal was founded in 1961 and is more concerned with promoting ideas of peace, using hoasca tea – a hallucinogenic drink containing only chacruna and caapi – to aid concentration in religious settings.

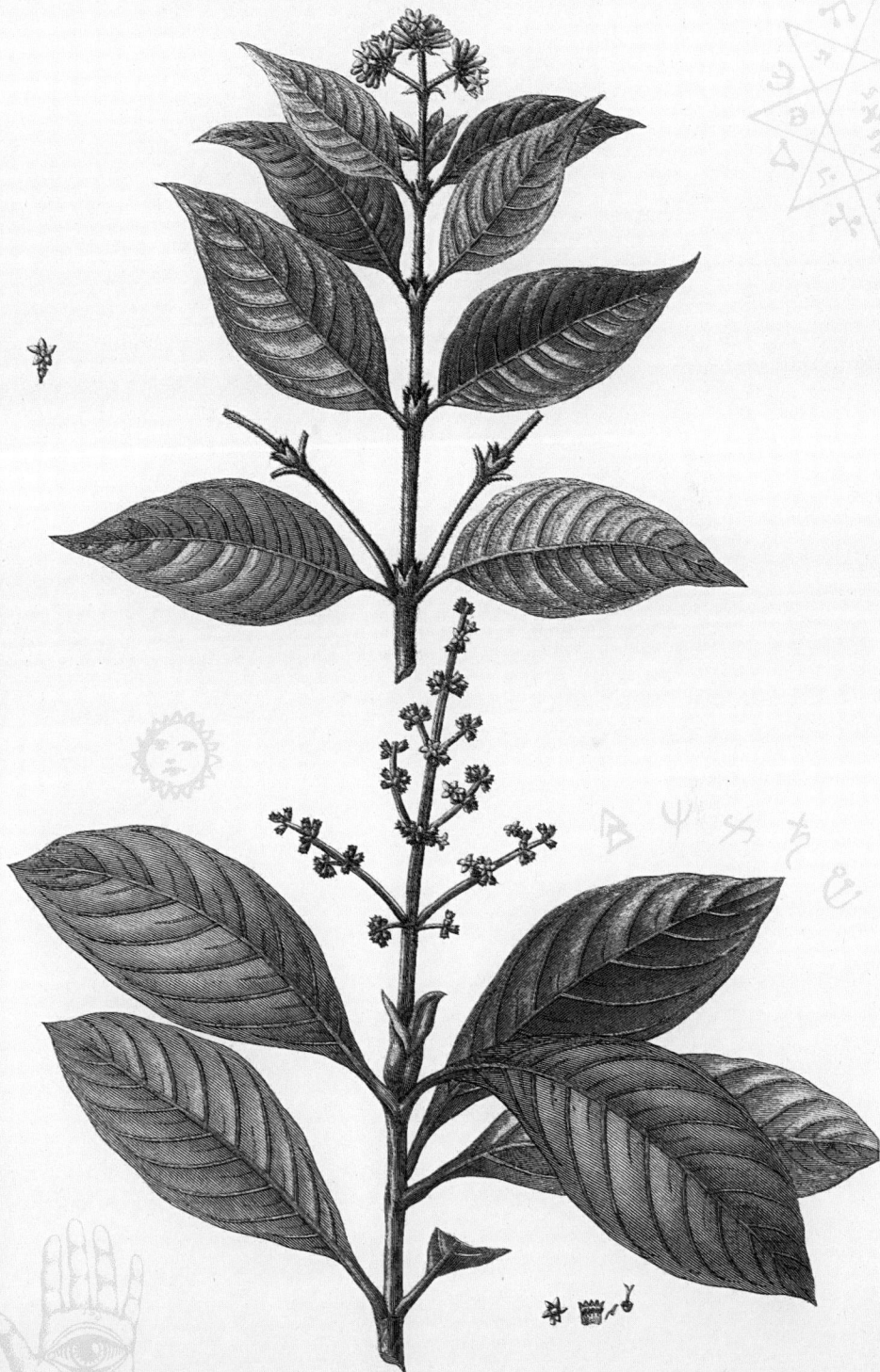

Ayahuasca

(including
Banisteriopsis caapi)

Ayahuasca is, for some, the latest in a long line of trendy
Western psychedelic fashions. For the indigenous Amazonian
peoples who have revered this teacher-drink for centuries, it
reveals nothing less than the meaning of life.

Confusingly, the word *ayahuasca* is sometimes used as a common name for *Banisteriopsis caapi*, a thick, woody rainforest vine with psychoactive compounds, one of the main ingredients in a drink of the same name.

The drink ayahuasca, whose dozens of local names include yajé, has as many recipes as practitioners. Every plant in the brew has its own story to tell, and its own lesson to teach, which may be learned by communing with the spirit world. Ingredients vary but always include one other plant: chacruna (*Psychotria viridis*, see p. 132). This is a shrubby plant in the coffee family, and contains a different psychoactive compound to that of *Banisteriopsis caapi*, but the two work together to produce an intense hallucinatory "journey". If caapi is the "essence" of the experience, chacruna allows you to "see" it.

Ayahuasca is no recreational wheeze. It is medicine, to be taken in deadly earnest, and the experience can be an ordeal. Preparation, both physically and mentally, takes time and effort as the freshly stripped bark is pounded, then boiled for hours by experienced *curanderos* (healers). Anyone may drink the bitter, sludgy brew, usually guided by the shaman, and the effects will be very personal.

The Shipibo-Conibo are an indigenous grouping of around 35,000 people living in the Peruvian Amazon, who believe that removing physical restrictions frees the mind to commune with the spirits, enabling it to cleanse and heal the body. Part of the preparation involves refraining from meat, alcohol, spices and sex for at least a week before.

The ceremony takes place by night, inside a thatched ancestral longhouse called a *maloca*. Depending on the group, dancing, music and *icaro* (chant) will play a major role. Nausea, dizziness and purging is very common. Everyone has their own vessel to use as they need; with the vomiting and diarrhoea they also rid themselves of evil. Six to twelve hours of vivid hallucinations are usually followed by deep sleep. Participants often

Opposite Shipibo Indian emboirdery of Ayahuasca
visions.

experience a sense of flying or being in touch with the earth and their ancestors. Some see green snakes, red jaguars or vivid geometrical shapes.

For the Shipibo, among others, ayahuasca is closely associated with La Madre, the primordial anaconda, whose skin bears the marks of all creatures, plants, humans and spirits, and who shares her wisdom with humans. An experienced healer may be able to diagnose someone's problems by feeling or smelling the air around them, or by visualizing their body covered in geometric markings. These are called *kené* and they are a fundamental part of Shipibo art, heavily based on the teachings of ayahuasca.

Featuring materials and pigments found in the rainforest, Shipibo beadwork, painting, embroidery, ceramics, textiles and body art is a representation of the various plants of power. Through the ingestion of ayahuasca, the *koshi* (energy) of the plant works with the human, who becomes a conduit for its spirit, and every piece is unique.

The British botanist Richard Spruce first encountered *Banisteriopsis caapi* in 1851, and ayahuasca has been a challenge for conventional science ever since. Isolating individual chemicals is one thing; working out how so many different compounds work together is something else. After centuries, traditional colonialist attitudes are now rapidly changing as scientists realize how much indigenous people have to teach them, but fundamental ideas of scientific "language" still need work. Rather than lumping together all plants of a certain kind as a single, Latin-based species, for example, indigenous people take a more subtle approach to classification, depending on a plant's age, soil conditions, or how much shade or moisture it has received. Individual plants will produce different

drinks, with different effects, something Western science, used to creating generic treatments for generic conditions, is slowly accommodating.

This is a tantalizing area of research, filled with opportunities in a world where conventional medicine is sometimes falling short, especially within the field of mental health. Anecdotally, the brew has reputedly helped with conditions ranging

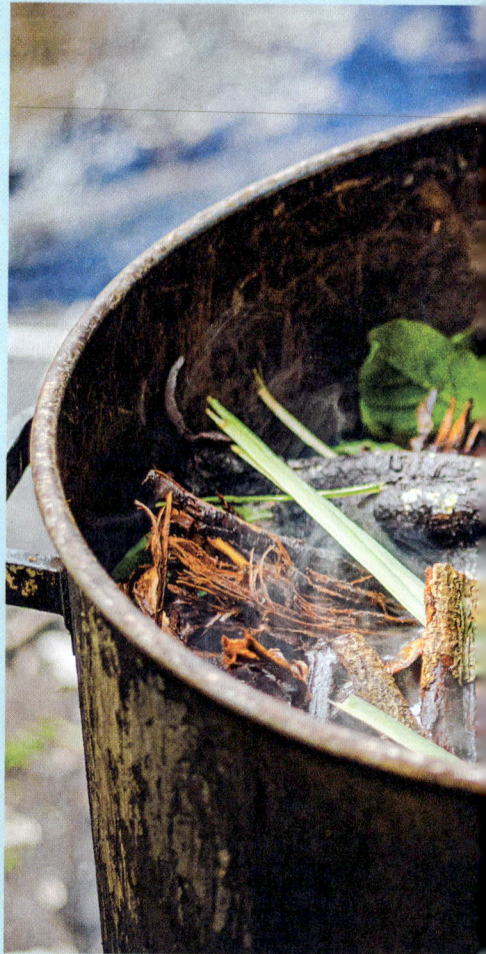

from depression and post-traumatic stress disorder to addiction and eating disorders, but not enough clinical trials have yet been carried out for any firm results.

Some people are not waiting. Following in the footsteps of Willaim S. Burroughs, Paul Theroux, Sting, Will Smith and a host of others, a new generation of ayahuasca tourists is turning to *Ayauasqueros* (ayahuasca shamans), either in their own countries or by travelling to the Amazon in search of some kind of truth. The authenticity of their experience will depend on whether the healers they trust are charlatans eager to fleece gullible gringos or the real deal.

Below Ayahuasca originated in South America and is used in spiritual ceremonies, healing and divination.

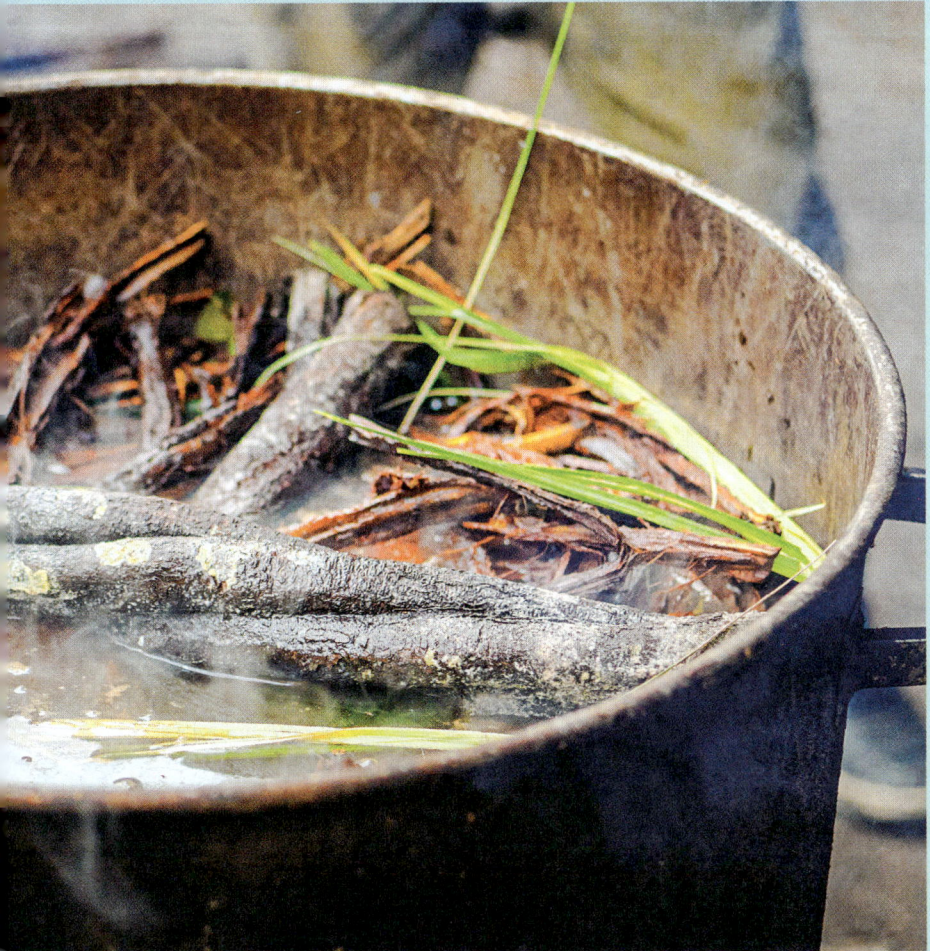

The Father of Ethnobotany:
Richard Evans Schultes 1915–2001

Mild-mannered Harvard professor in termtime, pith-
helmeted jungle explorer on vacation, Richard Evans Schultes
might have been the model for Indiana Jones – if he hadn't
treated his local scouts with so much respect and decency.

Schultes's legendary class – Biology 104, Plants and Human Affairs – would become a rite of passage for later students, though in 1933, when he took the module himself, he borrowed the slimmest book from the library so he would have time to write a paper on it and work his day job.

The book was *Mescal: The Divine Plant and its Psychological Effects*, by Heinrich Klüver, and it would change Schultes's life. Born in a poor area of Boston, he had entered Harvard on a scholarship and worked in the Botanical Museum to make ends meet. His paper was so impressive that museum director Oakes Ames funded Schultes's first field trip, to work on peyote cactus (see p. 183) with indigenous people in Oklahoma. The active word here is *with* – and working *with* people was, perhaps, Schultes's superpower, even beyond his calling for botany.

Probably the first westerner to truly understand that scientific endeavour was a two-way experience, Schultes insisted he never discovered any of the 24,000 plant specimens he brought back to the university. Instead, he patiently explained how the many indigenous peoples he lived with, undertook ceremonies with and collected with, had *shown* him not only the plant but how to interact with it.

Seeing a scribbled note in the university herbarium he next set off on a journey to Oaxaca, searching for the "mythical" magic mushrooms. He showed a few to his friend Albert Hofmann, who synthesized some, which would later be developed into a beta blocker.

Schultes was studying arrow poisons when Pearl Harbor was bombed in 1941. He reported for active duty but was sent back to the rainforest. Uncle Sam needed rubber, and the plantations in South East Asia had been seized by Japan. Schultes's task was to find an alternative. Living for more than 10 years with the Amazonian peoples, he conducted the first detailed studies of ayahuasca *and* found time to write about orchids and Harvard's extraordinary collection of glass flowers.

Back at Harvard, Schultes inspired a new generation of alternative ethnologists, but the man once described as "the most subversive person on Harvard Square" stayed away from the 1960s counterculture dramatics elsewhere on campus. His thoughts were far more radical. For all his extraordinary work in so many fields, perhaps the most important legacy of Richard Evans Schultes is that his was the first voice raised in alerting the world to the ecological peril of the Amazonian rainforest and its people.

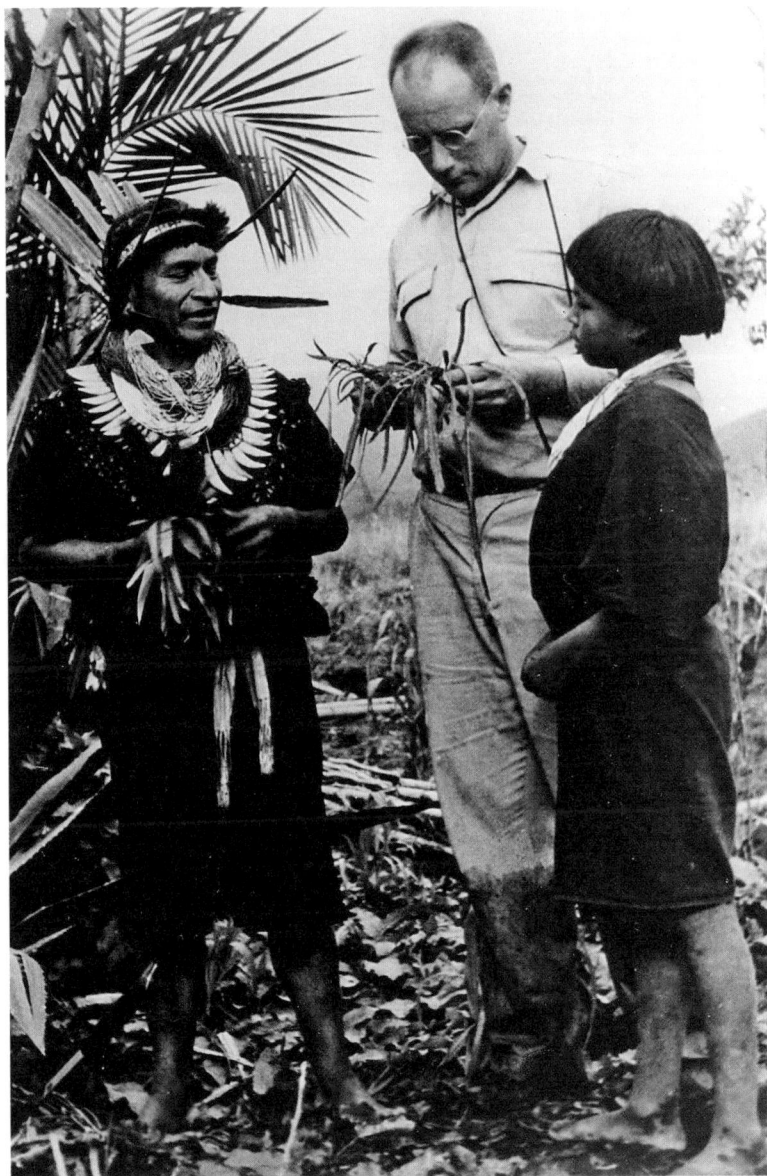

Above Dr Richard Evan Schultes was an American biologist considered to be the father of modern ethnobotany. Here he is pictured with two indiginous people in the Amazon in 1940.

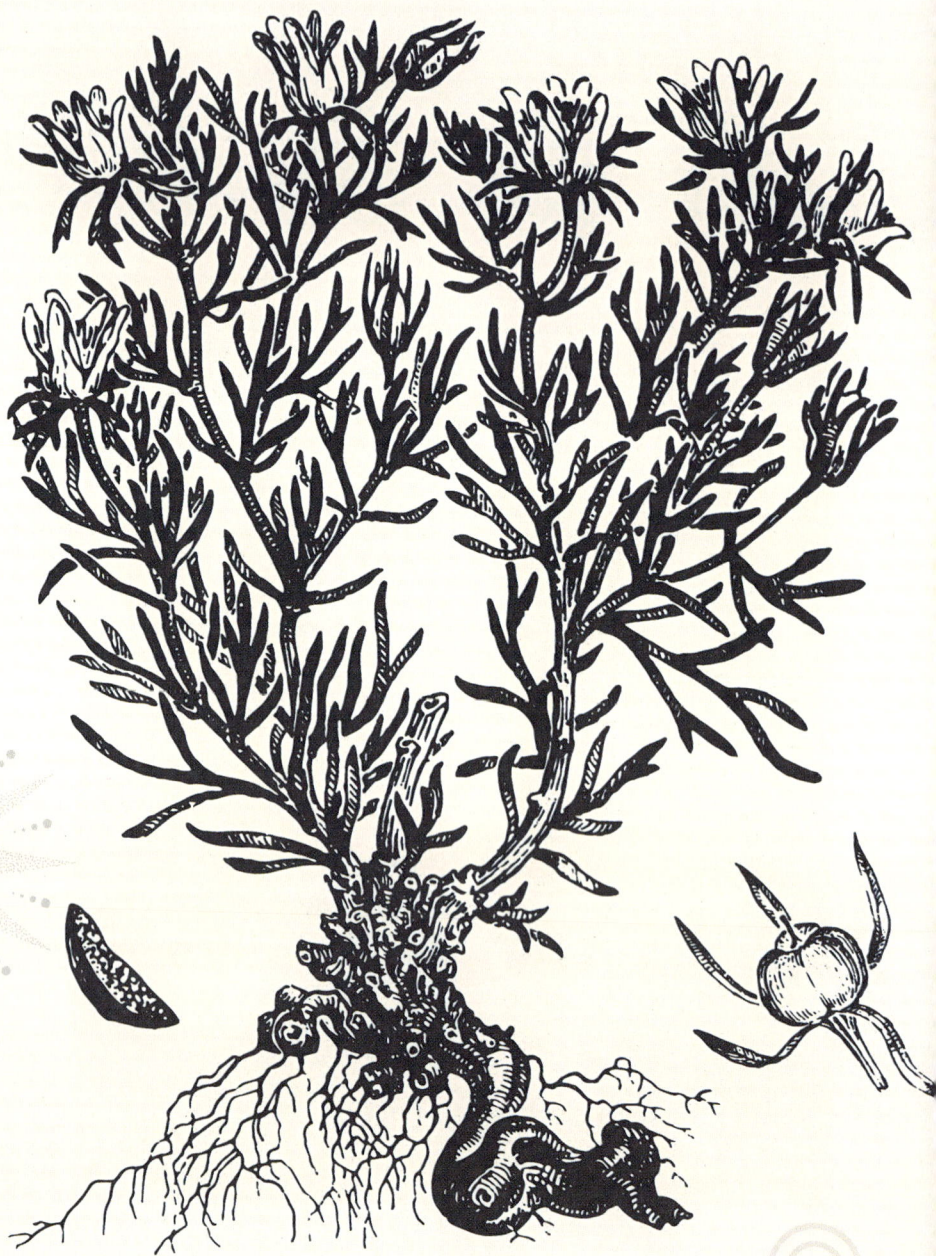

Syrian rue

Peganum harmala

While ayahuasca enjoys its moment in the sun, other intriguing herbs bask in the shade of relative anonymity. The seeds of Syrian rue contain similar chemicals to those found in the South American superstar. They just don't shout about it.

Growing wild from Mongolia and Manchuria through India and North Africa to the Middle East and Spain, Syrian rue (locally *harmala*) is unrelated to common rue (*Ruta graveolens*) but early scientists thought they looked similar. There is one very important difference between the two herbs, however: *Peganum harmala* contains hallucinogenic alkaloids.

The two major harmala compounds were among the first psychoactive substances ever isolated: harmaline by German chemist H. Göbel in 1841; harmine six years later by one J. Fritsch.

Like the caapi vine, harmala can, in high doses, have mild psychoactive effects, including weak visual illusions, but it has a far stronger impact when combined with other intoxicants, making it a classic ayahuasca *analogue* (alternative). Made into a drink with Jurema (*Mimosa tenuiflora*), the bitter-tasting (and foul-smelling) seeds can instil similar kaleidoscopic or firework-like hallucinations along with a sensation of movement or "travelling".

The alternative delights of harmala have been known since ancient times, and it has been suggested as the real-life *haoma*, the divine plant of Zoroastrianism and Persian mythology. Some have even linked it with the mythical *soma*, an ambrosia-like divine brew described in the ancient Indian Vedas. Scholars including Dioscorides, Galen and Avicenna were aware of harmala's mild psychoactive properties, but mainly proposed the herb's purgative qualities for more regular medicinal uses. The herb has played a profound, though non-hallucinogenic role in Middle Eastern life ever since.

The deep "Turkey red" dye of traditional Turkish carpets was originally extracted from harmala seeds, also ground for regular and tattoo ink, and while madder (*Rubia tinctorum*) is more popular today, some still cling to the old ways. Dried seed pods are hung around Moroccan houses and vehicles as talismans against evil djinn; Turkish and Iranian homes and cars enjoy similar protection from the evil eye. Known as *espand* in Iran, harmala seeds are burned at traditional Persian weddings to clear negative energy from the newly-weds' life together.

Syrian rue is toxic – it has been used as an abortifacient for centuries – but has recently spread to other countries where it is becoming a problem for livestock. Now an "invasive weed", this traditional enemy of evil has somehow become a notifiable alien in some states of the United States and China.

Chiricaspi

Brunfelsia grandiflora

The ayahuasca brew often includes many "satellite" ingredients, each of which adds its own special kick. *Brunfelsia grandiflora* is one of the drink's most common extras.

Science is good at isolating individual elements of a plant, but the sheer amount of work needed to investigate each compound means it can be slow to pinpoint effects when those elements are combined. This is bad enough in a single plant, which may contain many different chemicals, but complex recipes such as ayahuasca, with varying amounts of various substances, leave much research still to be done. Local knowledge, including names, can be invaluable in working out where to start.

There are around 49 species in the *Brunfelsia* genus, part of the nightshade (Solanaceae) family (see p. 164) and only a very few are known to have psychoactive properties. *Brunfelsia grandiflora* is known in the Quechua language as *chiricaspi* ("itching" or "cold" tree) thanks to the weird sensations brought on by drinking a brew made with it: a strange, tickling feeling as it goes down, followed by shivering and chills as it gets working.

A small tropical/subtropical tree thought to have originated in Central America, the chiricaspi has spread throughout northern South America, where it is used by many different communities to treat complaints ranging from rheumatism to snake bites.

Hallucinogenic in its own right, chiricaspi is more often included to intensify concoctions such as ayahuasca. According to the community, it may help diagnose disease (Cofán), induce purging (Shuar), aid hunting (Quechua), combat evil spirits or, as with the Siona people, check someone's paternity.

All parts of *Brunfelsia* are toxic, to both humans and animals (especially cats and dogs), so shamans only ingest it on its own when presented with a problem that cannot be solved through the usual channels. This may be taken as a brewed tea, or a cold drink made from soaked roots and stems. The Yabarana people of Venezuela first dry and then smoke it with tobacco.

The plant's many other common names, both local and Western, include "royal purple brunfelsia" and "kiss-me-quick". Confusingly, it is also sometimes known as "fever tree", thanks to another medicinal use (as a traditional treatment for ague) despite having no relation to *Vachellia xanthophloea*, the famous African fever tree immortalized by Rudyard Kipling or yet another "fever tree", *Cinchona*, which contains the anti-malarial compound quinine. *Brunfelsia*'s best-known nickname, "yesterday-today-tomorrow", comes from its highly floriferous nature; it blooms dark purple one day, pale lavender the next, and pure white the day after that. The tree is smothered in multicoloured blossom nearly all year round, providing flowers for people to wear or use as festival decorations.

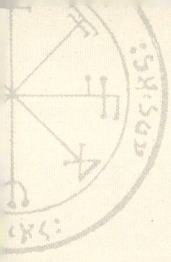

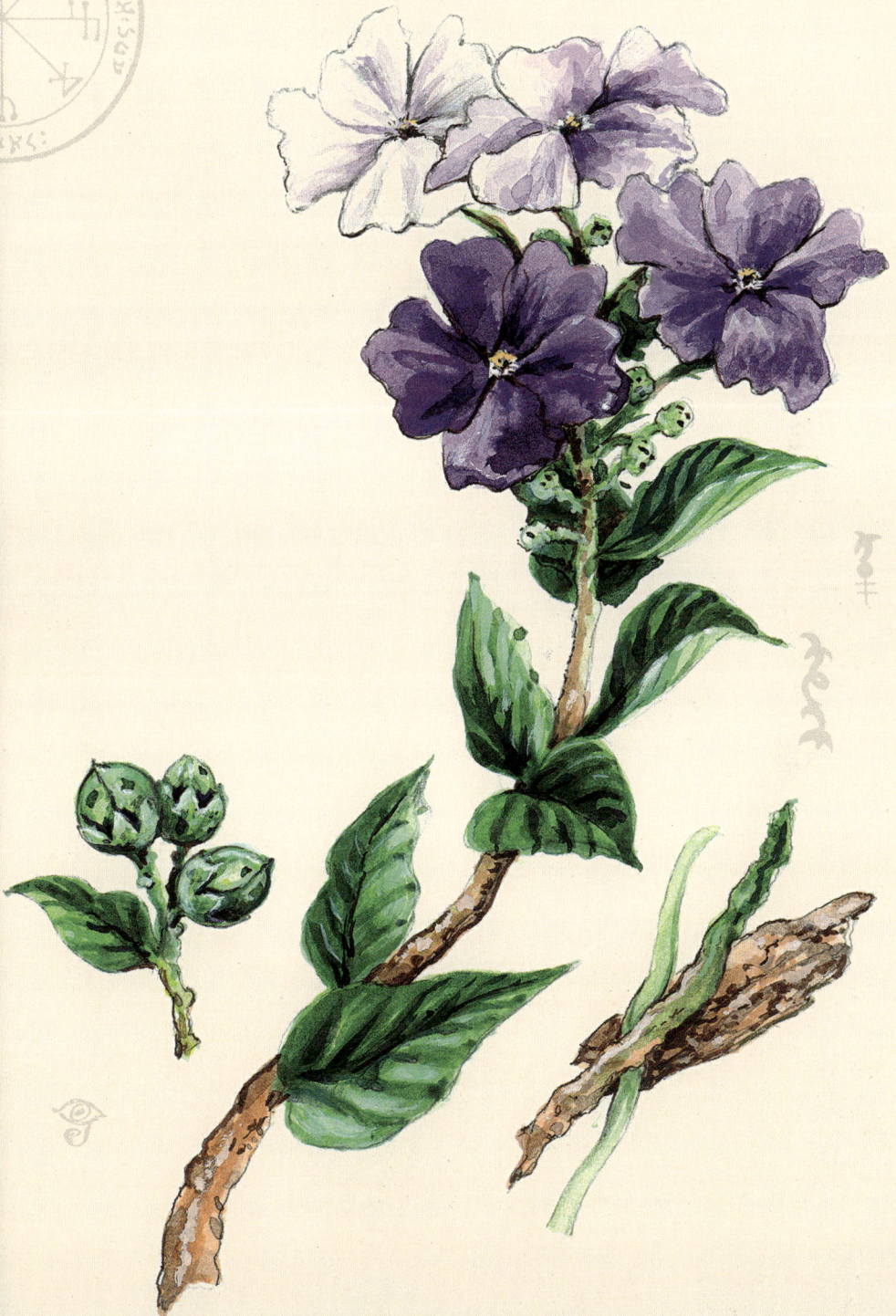

Chapter 8:
Art on Drugs

What do we mean by the idea of combining art and drugs? Do we mean art that depicts substance use, like the nineteenth-century fashion for painting absinthe drinkers? Work inspired by dreams experienced during a vision quest? Art made while using? Or are we more swayed by media gossip about individuals who write, paint, act or compose at nigh-on genius level but are better known by the public as users? All in their ways, are valid; all have been with us for as long as history can tell us.

Cosmic Designs

Kaleidoscopic images in saturated colour, combinations of the abstract and an almost archaic, figurative style appear in fine art and design across the 1960s. It can be difficult to separate the whole, roiling firmament into individual works.

A direct result of the hallucinogenic effects of psychedelic substances including psilocybin, peyote and ayahuasca alongside the ubiquitous LSD, such art is both comforting and challenging, the perfect expression of counterculture youth.

Practitioners resonated with previous movements, including Dada and Surrealism (Salvador Dalí famously experimented with mescaline, found in peyote and San Pedro cacti), but also looked to other media, including science fiction, experimental music and pulp novels, and often collaborated with other disciplines. Wes Wilson, Stanley Mouse, Alton Kelley, Rick Griffin and Bonnie MacLean were just a few of the leading San Francisco artistic community whose posters for the Fillmore music venue became iconic in themselves. Combing the intensely ornate typefaces and swirling lines of Art Nouveau, the anarchic influences of art movements from the early twentieth century and the driving guitar rock of their subjects, they churned out almost 300 disturbing, claustrophobic, almost unreadable but instantly recognizable posters for the likes of Jimi Hendrix, Santana, Jefferson Airplane and the Grateful Dead between 1965 and 1971.

Every aspect of 1960s culture would eventually bathe in psychedelic art, from album covers and onstage shows, to zines, murals, fashion, politics and even mainstream advertising. In the art world, all bets were off, from the pop art created by Roy Lichtenstein and Andy Warhol, both inspired by popular culture, to Bridget Riley's geometric op art via the happenings of performance art by figures such as Allan Kaprow, blurring the lines between disciplines. Comic books were suddenly taken seriously. Gilbert Shelton's *Fabulous Furry Freak Brothers* and its offshoot, *Fat Freddy's Cat*, both celebrated and lampooned '60s counterculture.

Not all such art was directly inspired by psychedelic drug use, of course. Art is always a product of its times, politics, mood and sensibilities. But the drugs helped.

In all this, the work of indigenous people was quietly forgotten. Few tourists on the hippie trail bothered to talk to the artists inspired by the entheogens they were so keen to try: the exquisite yarn paintings made by Huichol artists, depicting mythological figures from peyote vision-quests; or the sharply geometric, zigzag, piranha-teeth and spiderweb motifs used in Shipibo-Konibo art, directly inspired by journeys into ayahuasca.

In the 1980s and 1990s Colombian painter Luis Eduardo Luna founded the Usko-Ayar (Spiritual Prince) School of Amazonian painting, in the Peruvian city of Pucallpa, encouraging art that explored the traditional rituals of the vision quest. Similar movements appeared – and are appearing – across the region. Often figurative, but including abstract and geometrical elements, and combining traditional techniques with Western media and natural media, art by practitioners such as Pablo Amaringo is finally finding its place in the world.

Below Psychedelics inspired a type of art characterised by swirling patterns and bright colours.

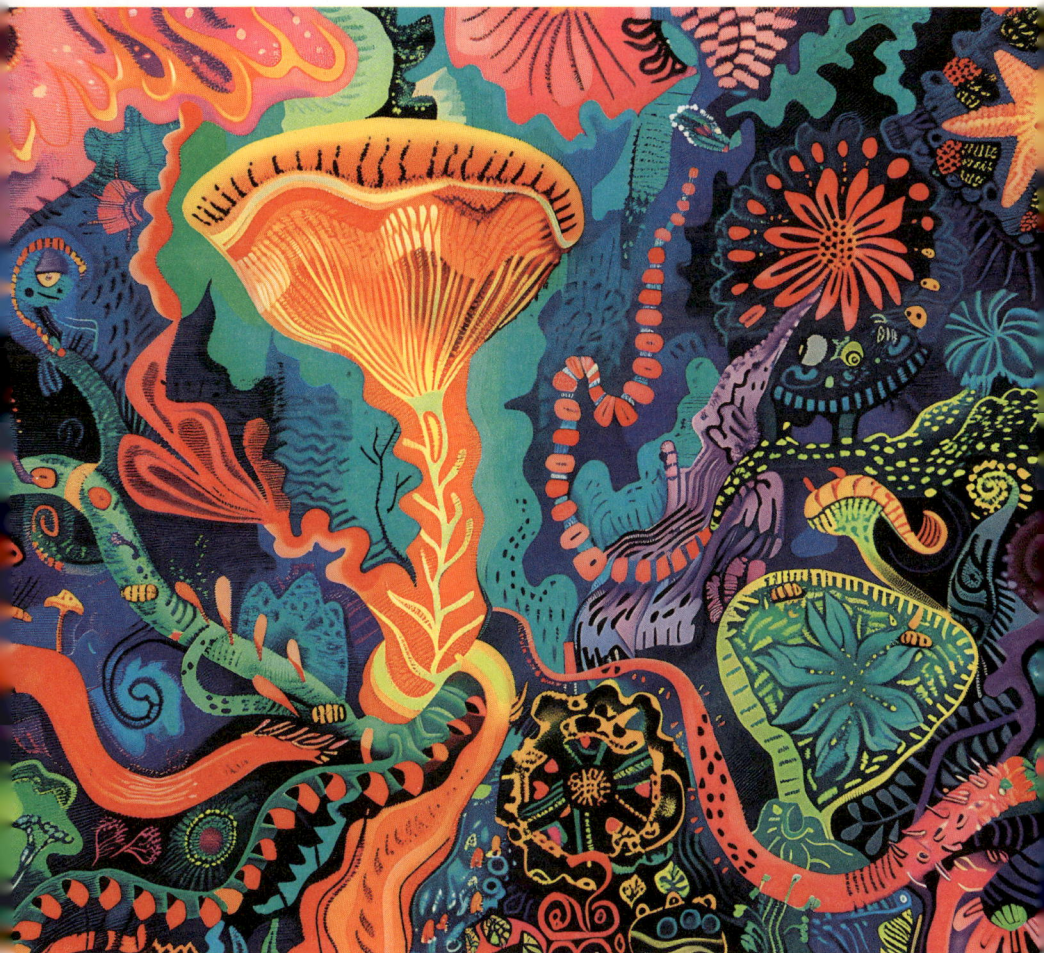

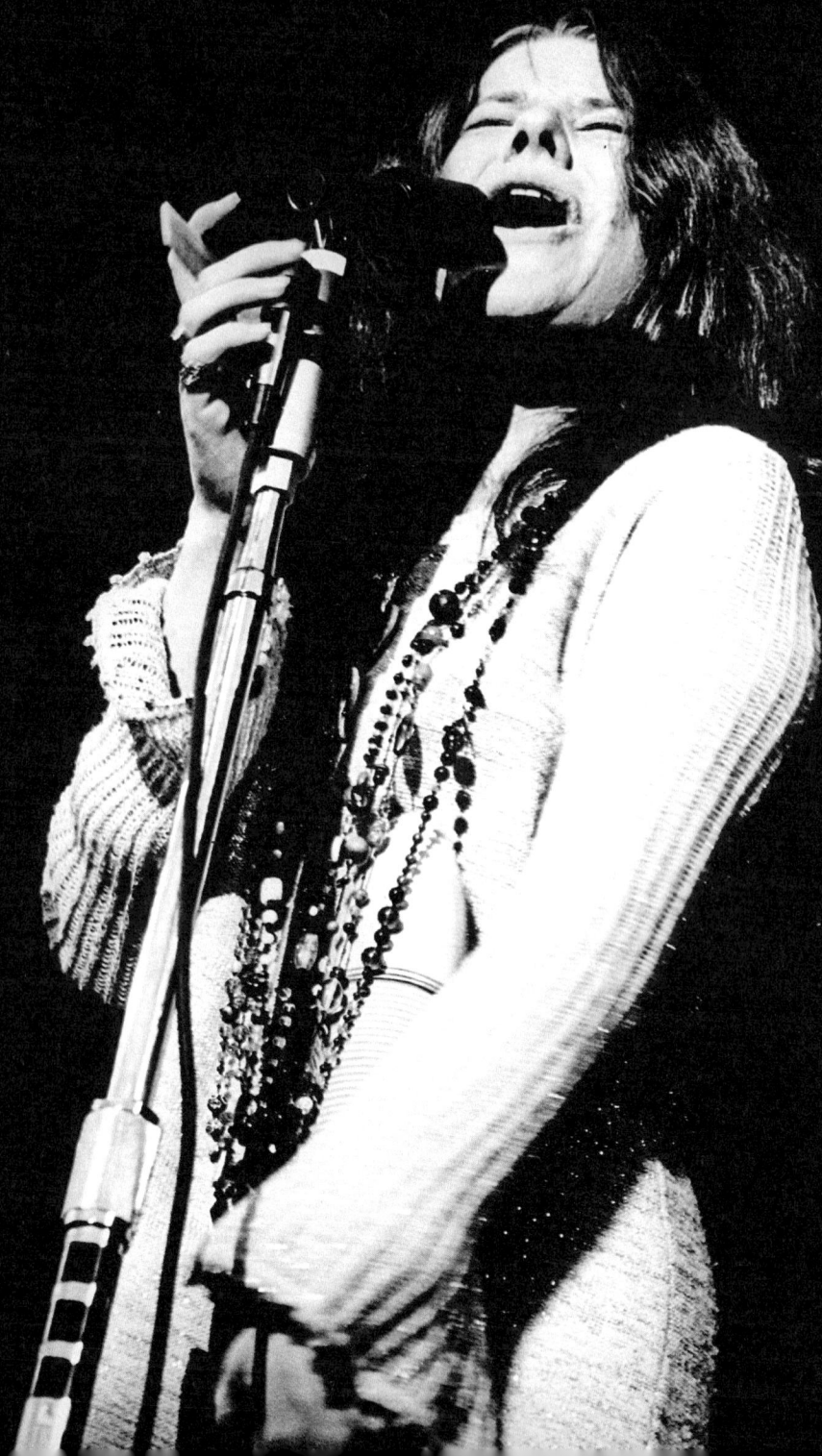

The Magical Mystery Tour

Sex & drugs & rock & roll have gone together since long
before Ian Dury was singing about them in 1977. Long before,
even, rock & roll was a thing.

The Great Migration saw six million African Americans move from the grinding poverty of the USA's rural southern states to relative poverty in the urban north, especially Chicago, New York, Detroit and Philadelphia. All four would become cradles for specifically Black styles of music, from blues to swing. Drugs were a crucial part of the scene, as a creative tool or simply as medicine, for body and soul, so it is unsurprising that songs about substances, coded in "jive talk", were almost universal among early jazz musicians. Louis Armstrong spent nine days in jail for smoking one of the joints he later celebrated in his 'Song of the Vipers' (1934), but his was just one of many "reefer songs", including Cab Calloway's cover of Fats Waller's 'Viper's Drag' (and his better-known 'Reefer Man', 1932) and the Harlem Hamfats' 'Weed Smoker's Dream' (1936), later reworded and recorded as 'Why Don't You Do Right?'. Stuff Smith's 1936 'If You're a Viper' is ostensibly about cannabis but also refers to cocaine, advising the listener to 'bust your conk on peppermint candy'. Even Ella Fitzgerald, the First Lady of Song, recorded the unequivocal 'Wacky Dust' in 1938.

There is a clear line from such music to more modern forms, including R & B (in both the old style of the 1940s and '50s and contemporary styles), hip-hop, rap and beyond. Marijuana is still celebrated, with the added dynamic of its being a cornerstone of the Rastafarian faith. Bob Marley argued passionately for cannabis as an expression of freedom. His former bandmember Peter Tosh went a step further, recording the album *Legalize It* in 1976.

Like its film equivalent, stoner music has a strong, if largely horizontal, following, though not much could follow the 63-minute, metal-inspired album *Dopesmoker*, recorded by the band Sleep in 1999. It's heavy stuff, but such music often has a comedic side, such as Afroman's 'Because I Got High' (2000) or Willie Nelson's 'Roll Me Up and Smoke Me When I Die' (2012) featuring Snoop Dogg, Kris Kristofferson and Jamey Johnson.

The Summer of Love – and the years immediately before it – spawned the music we commonly think of as psychedelic, not least because technology was (just about) keeping up with human imagination. Some bands revelled in the simplicity of folk music traditions. Scott McKenzie famously called America's youth to non-combatant arms, telling them to go to San Francisco wearing flowers in their hair. Others were seduced by high tech, including work pioneered by the Brotherhood Of Light, a collective of multimedia stage technicians. Strobe lighting, visuals pulsating like lava lamps

Opposite Janis Joplin, the Queen of Psychedelic Soul, pictured in 1967.

and electronic sound machines created spacey live shows. Experimental recording techniques including distortion, guitar tremolo (aka "whammy bar"), multitracking and switching between left and right channels on new stereo equipment, made for a psychedelic home experience courtesy of the latest invention: hi-fi. Wildly imaginative album covers and posters completed the package. Bands such as the Grateful Dead, Cream and the Velvet Underground, along with artists like Janis Joplin, Dr. John and even Bob Dylan after his conversion to electricity, pushed at the boundaries of music. Jefferson Airplane's acid-tinged *After Bathing at Baxters* and the eponymous debut album by the Doors, both released in 1967, join the Grateful Dead's 16-track epic *Aoxomoxoa* (1960) and Jimi Hendrix's virtuoso *Electric Ladyland* (1968) as some of rock's all-time greatest albums. Even TV pop funsters the Monkees got into the act with 'The Porpoise Song', as they battled studio executives for control over their own music.

At the forefront of innovation since the early '60s, the Beatles, alongside pioneering producer George Martin, were always ahead of any game being played. John Lennon called *Rubber Soul* (1965) the band's "pot album"; the following year's *Revolver* and 1967's *Sgt. Pepper's Lonely Hearts Club Band* were the real psychedelic deal, a swirling soup of LSD-fused hits. The group's involvement with Eastern spiritual traditions also saw them experimenting with "exotic" instruments. The sitar would become a genre mainstay. The same year the band aimed to break out further: *Magical Mystery Tour*, a crazy, trippy TV extravaganza juxtaposing everyday 1960s Britain with the psychedelic world the lads from Liverpool now inhabited, didn't really work as a concept, not least because British television was still largely black and white, but the album has since become a cult classic.

Music marched on. Songs about, or written using, substances were omnipresent. Sometimes it was coded, as in Lou Reed's 'Perfect Day' (1972). The Beatles' 'Got to Get You into My Life' (1966) was, Paul McCartney would later explain, "an ode to pot". Usually, though, they were more explicit: Eric Clapton's 'Cocaine' (1976); the Velvet Underground's 'Heroin' (1967); Pink Floyd's 'Comfortably Numb' (1980); James Brown's 'King Heroin' (1972); Marianne Faithfull and the Rolling Stones's 'Sister Morphine' (1969); and Black Sabbath's 'Sweet Leaf' (1971).

Substance use, especially in "softer" form such as marijuana, is marginally less shocking these days, so there are fewer examples of songs about it. But with recordings such as 'Ulysses' (Franz Ferdinand, 2009), 'Can't Feel My Face' (the Weeknd, 2015) and 'D.R.E.A.M.' (Miley Cyrus, 2019) we can be sure of one thing: while sex and rock & roll exist, the drugs will be there too.

Opposite A 1980s USA Jimi Hendrix poster. His song 'Purple Haze' is often interpreted as referring to a psychedelic experience.

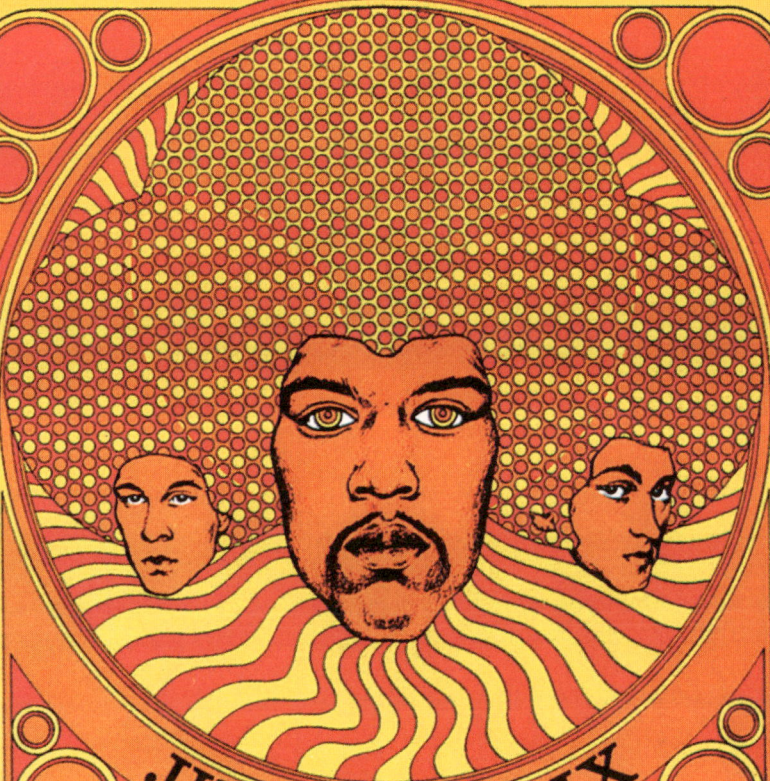

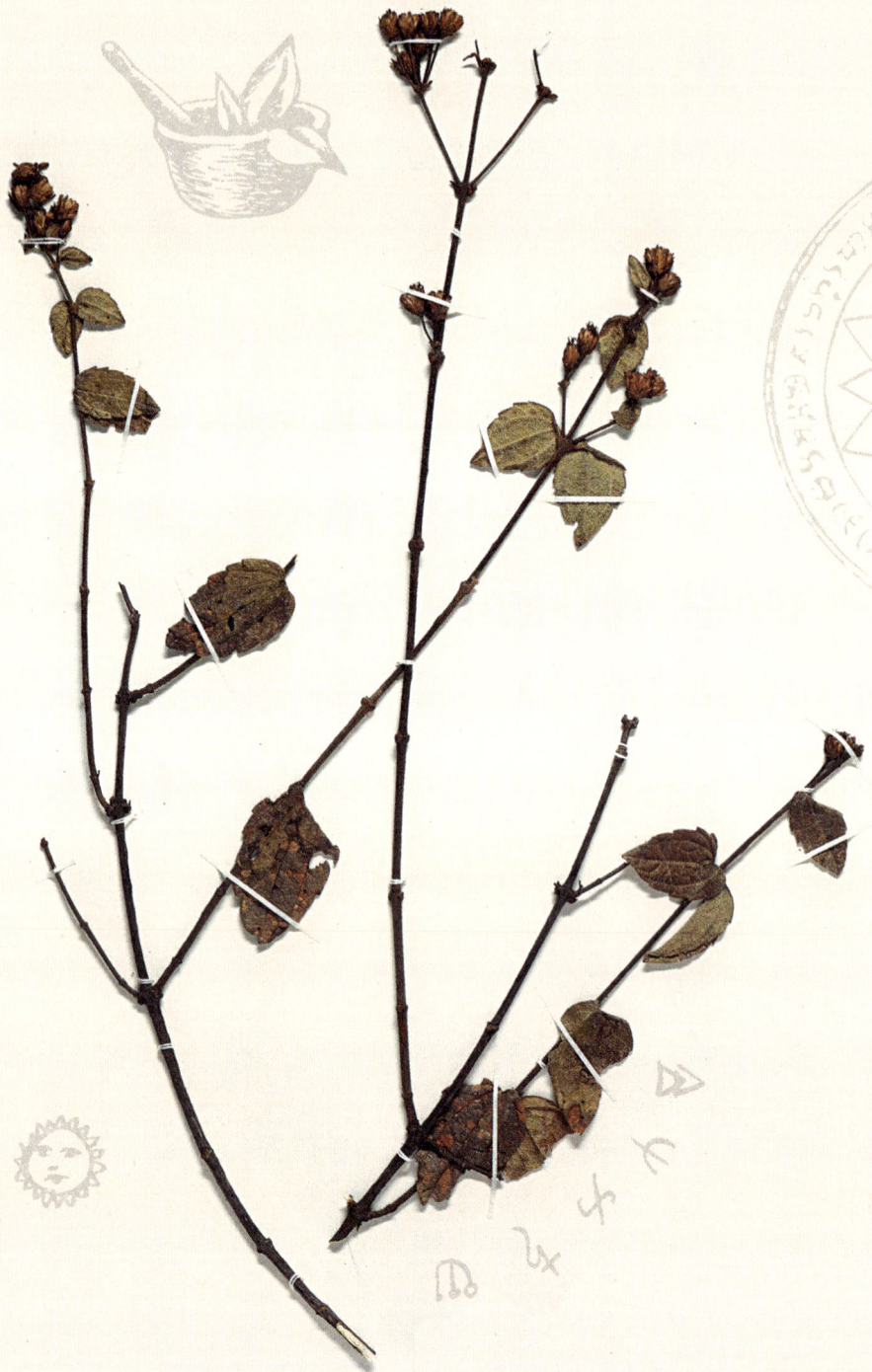

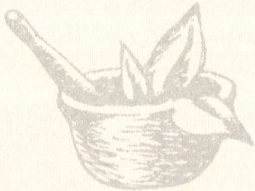

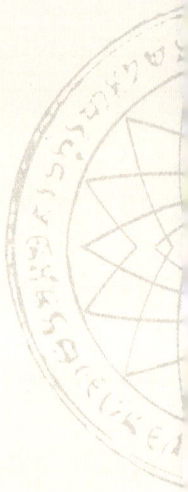

Mexican dream herb

Calea ternifolia

Every community that uses Mexican dream herb has a
different name for it, but they all include one word: "bitter".

Whether they call it *tam huñi* (bitter gum), *poop taam ujts* (white bitter herb) or *zacatl chichic* (from the Nahuatl for "bitter grass"), no one is pretending it tastes good, but its uses, both medicinally and spiritually, are revered.

Calea ternifolia (formerly *zacatechichi*, from the Nahuatl) is native to Central America, though it is also found in Costa Rica and southern Texas. It is part of the Asteraceae family which includes sunflowers and daisies, but its small, white, "fluffy" flowers and unremarkable leaves do not make it a natural addition to the ornamental garden. For the shamans of the Chontal people of Oaxaca, however, it is a sacred plant bearing *thlepelakano*: leaves of God.

Several indigenous cultures use the herb medicinally, as a traditional remedy for complaints such as stomach ache, diarrhoea and fevers; it is also sometimes used as an insecticide, but only the Chontal use the Aztec dreaming herb as a divinatory tool.

The leaves are dried, then made into a tea. The drinker afterwards smokes a cigarette made from more dried leaves, inducing drowsiness followed by sleep, and encouraging lucid dreams. Some report a heightened awareness of their heart and pulse; larger doses can incite hallucinations. Shamans use the herb to divine medical or other problems; others may use it for meditation and a sense of tranquillity.

There have been studies made of the dreaming herb's effects, some more scientific than others, suggesting an enhanced state of perception and creativity after taking the herb, and that it can cause nausea and vomiting, or interfere with other drugs. However, not enough is yet known about the plant's scientific composition to be completely sure of its powers or possible contraindications.

One of *Calea*'s biggest American fans is David Woodard, the avant-garde artist and composer. He is best known for his work with Gysin and Sommerville's psychedelic Dreamachine, a stroboscopic light device that fits on a record turntable and produces visions when "viewed" with closed eyes, but Woodard is also famous for his requiems for dead wildlife and notorious for his "prequiems" for soon-to-be-dead humans. He successfully grew the plant at his home in San Francisco in the 1990s, and celebrated with a motet, *Calea Zacatechichi*, composed for *Infernal Proteus, a Musical Herbal*. This multimedia project, released by indie label Ajna Offensive in 2002, involved 40 artists from 13 countries who created work based on mind-altering plants. Woodard recorded the piece with a children's choir from an all-Hispanic junior high school in East Los Angeles, grateful that no one ever asked him what *Calea zacatechichi* actually was...

Reefer Madness: Hollywood on Drugs

The motion picture you are about to witness may startle you.
It would not have been possible otherwise to sufficiently
emphasize the frightful toll of the new drug menace which is
destroying the youth of America...

So run the opening credits of kitsch classic *Tell Your Children*, originally made in 1936 by a church group, warning parents of the horrors of cannabis but later purchased by Dwain Esper, whose exploitation B-movies included *Sex Maniac, Narcotic Racket* and *The Strange Loves of Adolf Hitler*. Esper added some saucy scenes and reissued the film as *Reefer Madness*, cashing in on a new puritanism that had spawned both the 1937 Marihuana Tax Act, effectively outlawing cannabis, and the Motion Picture Production Code, a "voluntary" set of moral guidelines dreamed up by chairman William Harrison Hays.

Pre-Code Hollywood was as relaxed about portraying drugs as it was about sex, nudity, violence and alcohol. An early example saw Douglas Fairbanks's cocaine-addicted sleuth Coke Ennyday (no, really) camping up the 1916 Sherlock Holmes parody *The Mystery of the Leaping Fish*. Later, drugs featured in various genres, including melodrama, as with Dawn O'Day's no-specific dependency in *Three on a Match* (1932), and even musicals. 'Sweet Marijuana' is a Busby Berkeley-style production number complete with chaps in satin flares and sombreros strumming guitars while topless ladies

Opposite A film poster from 1955 advertising *The Man with the Golden Arm*. The film was controversial on release as it explores the then-taboo subject of drug addition.

coyly peep from cactus flowers (cannabis...peyote, all the same, thing really...) in *Murder at the Vanities* (1934), a picture that just sneaked in as the Code started raining on Hollywood's parade.

All was not entirely lost. Under the Methods of Crime section defined by the Production Code Authority (PCA), "drug traffic should not be presented in any form" but drug *use* only came under the "be careful" category. As long as they were shown to be A Bad Thing, drugs could still appear – hence Dwain Esper's ability to show *Reefer Madness* under the banner of "moral guidance". Lurid magazines helped fuel the public panic with more scaremongering. *Hush-Hush*, Danny de Vito's fictional scandal sheet in *L.A. Confidential* (1997), is unashamedly based on the real *Confidential* magazine.

What happened on-screen did not reflect what was going on behind the camera. Many Golden Age actors were routinely given "pep" pills to wake them up, and "sleeping tablets" to bring them down again. *Confidential* loved nothing better than busting starlets, especially when they moved on to worse substances, and there were tragedies, none sadder than the death of Judy Garland. They still happen, most recently with the tragic loss of Matthew Perry; it is more positive to concentrate on the stars who have turned the corner, such as Robert Downey Jr. and Drew Barrymore.

FRANK SINATRA · ELEANOR PARKER · KIM NOVAK

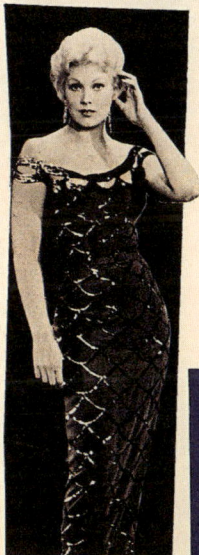

THE MAN WITH THE GOLDEN ARM

A FILM BY OTTO PREMINGER

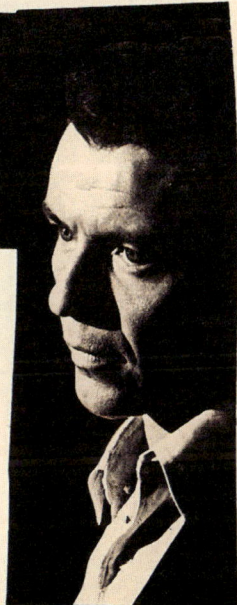

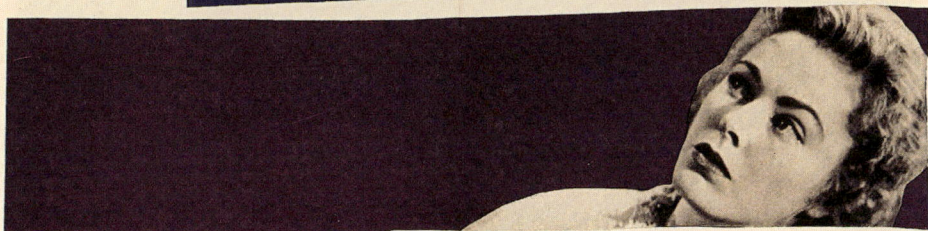

With Arnold Stang, Darren McGavin, Robert Strauss, John Conte, Doro Merande, George E. Stone, George Mathews, Leonid Kinskey, Emile Meyer, Shorty Rogers, Shelly Manne, Screenplay by Walter Newman & Lewis Meltzer, From the novel by Nelson Algren, Music by Elmer Bernstein, Produced & Directed by Otto Preminger, Released by United Artists

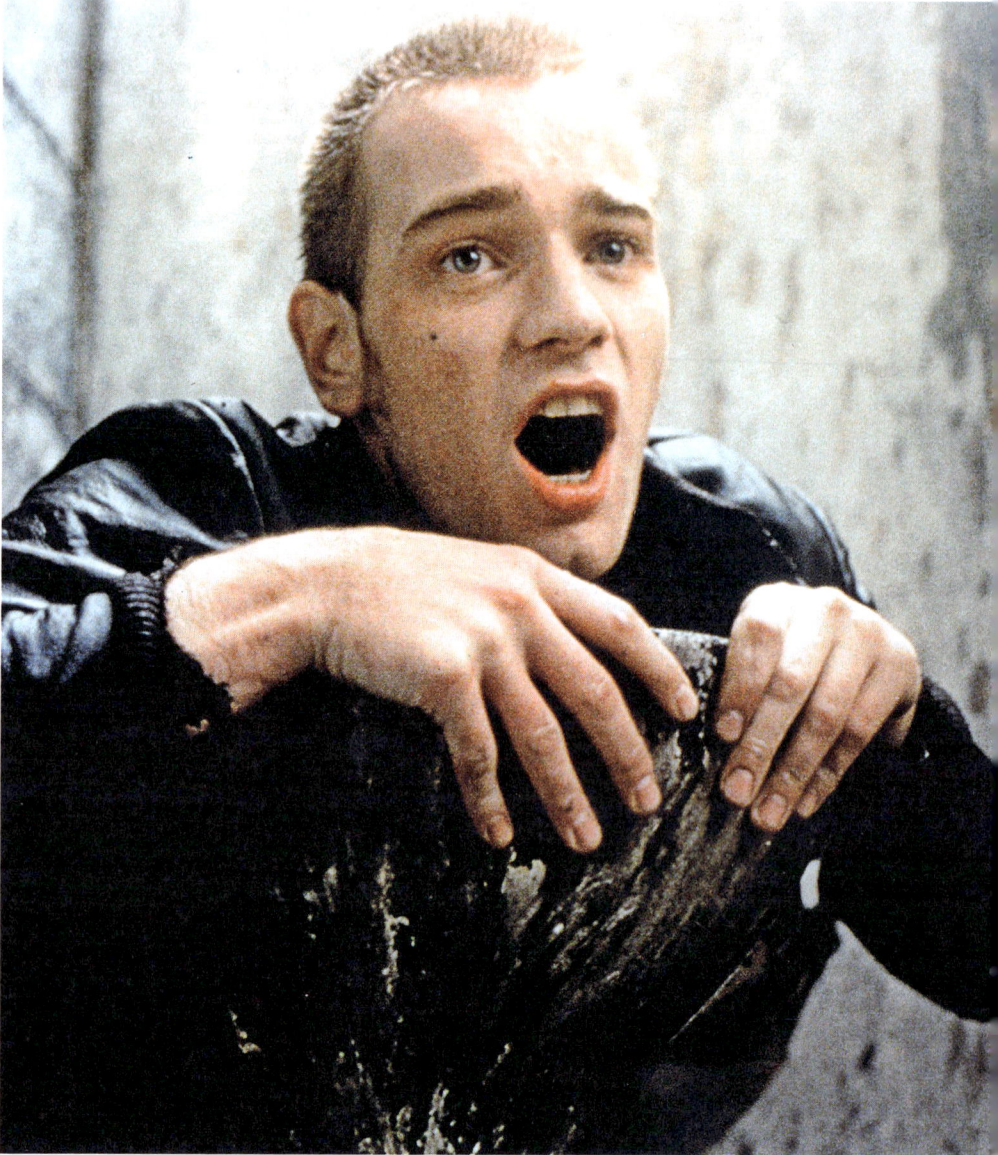

By the 1950s, the Code was beginning to show signs of strain. The script for Otto Preminger's *The Man with the Golden Arm* (1955), where former teen heartthrob Frank Sinatra shot up with heroin, then went through the consequences, was, unsurprisingly, rejected. Privately, however, Preminger was encouraged to release the film anyway, which he did, forcing a rethink by the PCA. By the 1960s the censor's lock was picked.

"Psychedelic" movies may involve peyote – for example, *Beyond the Valley of the Dolls* (1970), *Young Guns* (1988), *The Doors* (1991) and even *Beavis and Butt-Head Do America* (1996) – or psilocybin, as with *Natural Born Killers* (1994), but they are more likely to feature the synthetic LSD. Perhaps surprisingly, however, given the artistic possibilities of psychedelia, Hollywood appears to be far more interested in straight-up hard drugs. This may have something to do with another cinema obsession, crime. Many mainstream drug-based movies swirl around the supply chain of cocaine, heroin and anything else the characters can lay their hands on, but often also show the traders sampling their own wares. *Easy Rider* (1969) sees Dennis Hopper and Peter Fonda taking off on now-iconic motorbikes after a cocaine deal, giving a whole new meaning to the phrase *road trip*. Al Pacino's Tony Montana both sells and uses cocaine in *Scarface* (1983), signalling his downfall, while the real-life gangster Henry Hill

only begins his descent with the mob when he starts dealing coke in Martin Scorsese's film of his life, *Goodfellas* (1990). Recently, some intriguing films about drug dealing have shown a more nuanced side to drug sales, including the unflinching Spanish film *Maria Full of Grace* (2004), which follows a 17-year-old trying to break away from a life of drudgery while becoming embroiled with a Bogotá drug cartel. A less-than-glamorous take on heroin may also be found in the black comedy *Trainspotting* (1996); the even darker *The Wolf of Wall Street* (2013) is based on the coke-fuelled memoirs of boiler-room criminal and former stockbroker Jordan Belfort.

In the 1970s, *Reefer Madness* found a new, post-ironic audience within "stoner" movies, a comedy sub-genre usually but not always based around marijuana. The films of Cheech Marin and Tommy Chong grew out of the pair's stand-up routines, while *Fear and Loathing in Las Vegas* (1998) was spawned from Hunter S. Thompson's novel of the same name. Few knew, at first, what to make of the Dude, anti-hero of Joel and Ethan Cohen's crime comedy *The Big Lebowski* (1998), but Jeff Bridge's dishevelled performance – not entirely unlike those of the great Raymond Chandler gumshoes – has since gained "classic" status. It is preserved in the Film Registry of the Library of Congress as "culturally significant". Whatever would Will Hays have made of that?

Opposite In *Trainspotting*, Renton, played by Ewan McGregor, is deeply immersed in the drug scene in Edinburgh. The film charts his attempt to clean up and get out.

Kava

Piper methysticum

"Pacific elixir" has been drunk across the South Sea Islands
for centuries to invoke spirits, revere ancestral guardians,
aid decision-making, welcome visitors and amicably
settle disputes.

Kava (sometimes kava kava) is made from the "narcotic pepper", which has many cultivars, each with its own specific psychoactive properties. The name *Piper* comes from the Latin for "pepper" – it is a member of the Piperaceae or pepper family – and *methysticum* means "intoxicating". The tough rhizomes were once chewed first by young people with good teeth, before being combined with coconut milk and strained into ornate bowls. Kava is a hypnotic narcotic, rather than hallucinogenic, producing a feeling of well-being.

The plant enjoys several origin stories across the many islands. In Fiji, where it is the national drink, Degei the creator god was searching for his lost friend, a hawk called Turuwaka, but found only her abandoned nest. He cared for the two eggs inside, which hatched as the first man and woman. He gave them two special gifts: vuga (*Metrosideros collina*), an evergreen tree with bright flowers, and kava.

A Tongan tale tells of a couple living on a barren island, who sacrificed their only daughter when they had nothing to give a visiting king. Two plants grew on her grave, the sugar cane and kava. In a similar story from Vanuatu a boy accidentally kills his sister while protecting her honour. He mourns every day, then notices a mouse nibbling a plant on her grave, which drops dead. Wishing to see his sister again, the boy eats some himself, but instead feels relief and peace.

A different kind of relief came to women on the same island, where it is said two sisters were foraging wild yams in the forest. Squatting by the river to clean the vegetables, one of them was surprised when a stalk from a kava plant reached into her vagina, causing a very pleasant sensation. The sisters brought the plant home, and tended it secretly. Eventually they offered some to the menfolk who had been drinking a brew from wild kava that caused headaches. The story does not relate how much detail the sisters included in their tale of discovery.

Less saucily, Hawaiian mythology tells us that Loa, the legendary chief and explorer, brought kava back from his travels, where it became a drink for royalty and *kahunas* (important people) and a worthy offering for the gods, though others say it was found by the gods themselves. In large quantities, kava's euphoric effects can produce stupor, and in the 1980s "killer kava" or "the zombie drink" became a problem among Australian aboriginal communities. It has also recently been linked to liver damage and is therefore banned in some countries.

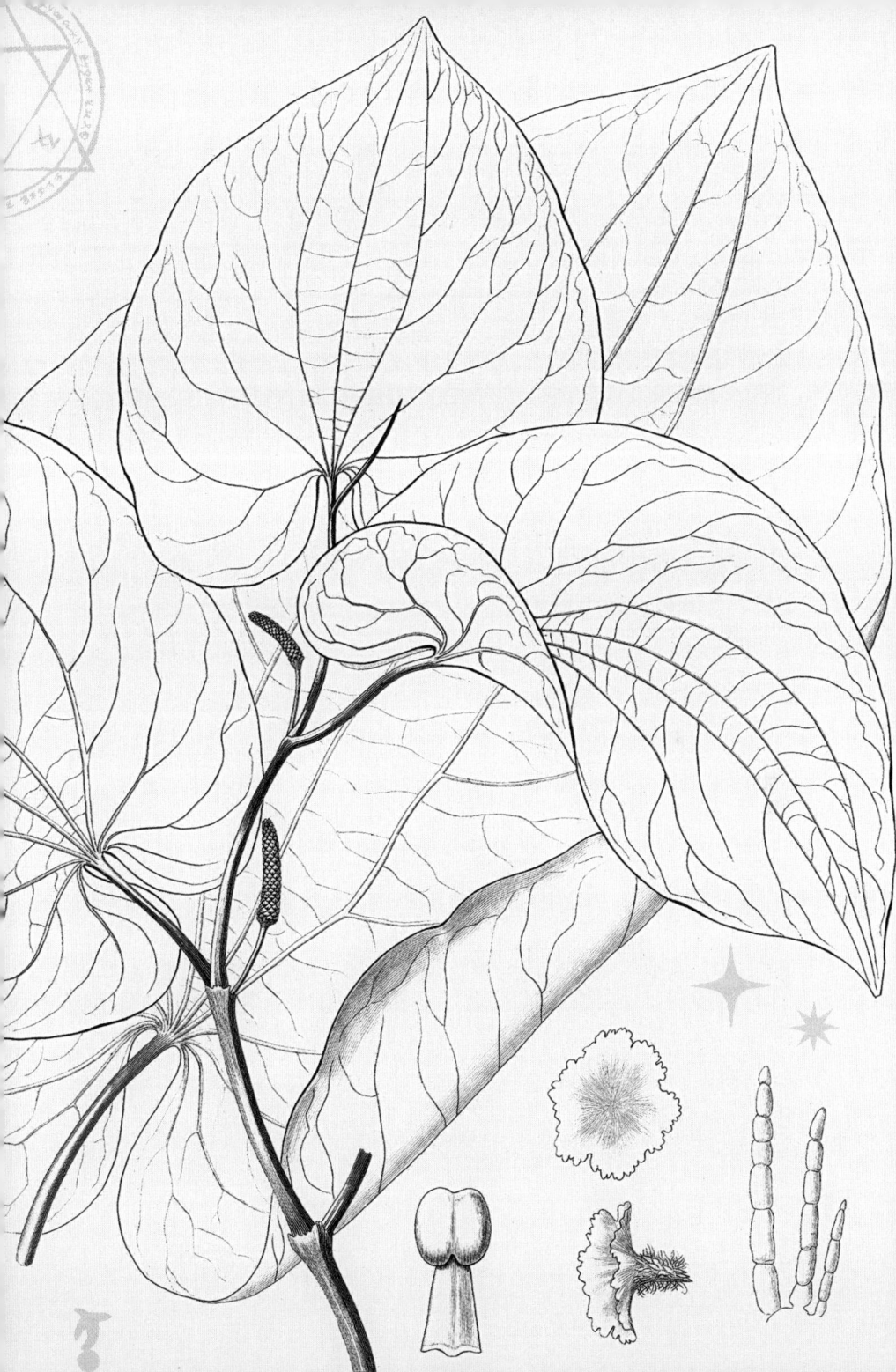

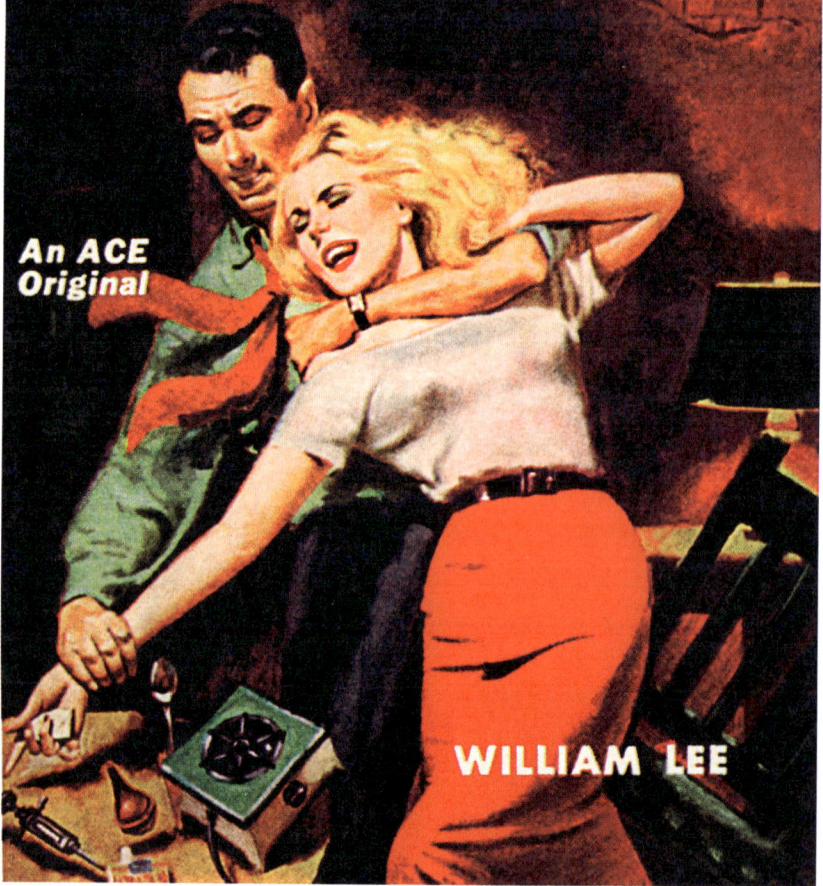

Above *Junkie* (1953) explores drug addiction,
including grotescque descriptions and imagery
of hallucinations.

Doors of Perception:
Literature of Substance(s)

Thomas de Quincy's *Confessions of an English Opium-Eater*
started a genre of writing about drugs as self-examination
which continues to this day, but substances appear in all forms
of the written word, both fact and fiction.

You could argue it goes back to at least Shakespeare. What is that blue herb Puck drips into Bottom's eyes in *A Midsummer Night's Dream*? The caterpillar's mushroom in *Alice's Adventures in Wonderland* (1865) is not psilocybin-like and the mysterious cake has currants, not cannabis, but this did not stop Jefferson Airplane writing a psychedelic anthem, 'White Rabbit', about Alice's otherworldly experiences.

Opium was a big deal in literature of the late nineteenth and early twentieth centuries. Conan Doyle's Sherlock Holmes in "The Man with the Twisted Lip" (1891), Agatha Christies' Hercule Poirot in "The Lost Mine" (1923), and Hergé's Tintin in *The Blue Lotus* (1936) are just three classic detectives who found themselves investigating the crime writer's favourite venue, the opium den. Drug use remains a popular theme in fiction, including the cocaine-fuelled hedonism of Jay McInerney's *Bright Lights, Big City* (1984) and the heroin haze of Irvine Welsh's Edinburgh-based fable, *Trainspotting* (1993).

During the 1950s and '60s, however, the real-life experiences of writers experimenting with psychedelic substances led to a new set of blended literary formats. William S. Burroughs's first novel *Junkie* (1953) and Aldous Huxley's autobiographical *The Doors of Perception* (1954), with its follow-up *Heaven and Hell* (1956), proved seminal. The style, ostensibly autobiographical while blurring reality with the imagined, released artists from the previous constraints of genre, allowing non-fiction to consort with postmodernism, poetry, confessional writing, science, psychiatry, fantasy, religious text, even comedy. Psychedelia was ripe for multimedia collaboration. Burroughs, for example, would inspire Canadian painter Brion Gysin to work on the Dreamachine (see p. 153), a bizarre, stroboscopic mechanical trip fashioned from flickering lights and a record player.

The agility of the psychedelic mind led to literary crossover too. There is the dystopian science fiction of Philip K. Dick's *A Scanner Darkly*, published in 1977, when 1994 was far enough away to be "the future". The angry comedy of Lenny Bruce. Hunter S. Thompson's ultra-subjective, gonzo journalism. Ralph Steadman's anarchic illustrations for Thompson's 1971 *Fear and Loathing in Las Vegas*, written in the gonzo style – a blend of autobiography, fiction, road trip, general mind blow and cartoon.

Modern writers may (or may not...) have moved on from using psychedelic substances to fuel their work, but we all benefit from the freedom bequeathed to us by the 1960s psychonauts after their own, very personal journeys into space.

Chapter 9:
The Hexing Herbs

A pointy hat. A black cat.
A cauldron. All classic
stereotypes associated with
Western witchcraft, yet nothing
beats the ultimate witch cliché:
broomstick flying. Better known
by their old English name
besom, brooms have been the
transport option of choice for
people accused of sorcery
since the Middle Ages, but they
couldn't just ride any old stick.
Enter the hexing herbs…

Solanaceae

Deliriants disorientate and confuse the body, often inducing hallucinations and the sensation of flying. Some affect the memory; the user may later have little or no recollection of their experience. The best-known, denounced as putative ingredients for the legendary 'flying ointment', are all to be found in the Solanaceae family.

The first-known picture of flying witches – one on a broom, the other on a plain stick – is an illumination from the 1451 manuscript *Le Champion des Dames*. The concept may have been metaphorical, but that did not stop the Church from taking it literally. The earliest accused broomstick-rider was Guillaume Edelin, a French priest arrested in 1453 after criticizing the Church's attitude to witchcraft. Edelin was tortured but, after a "confession", only imprisoned for life.

The notion of a "flying ointment" used by witches at so-called Black Sabbaths slowly grew to histrionic proportions during the medieval and early modern period. Formed of a variety of plants and fungi, the ointment was allegedly rubbed onto mucus membranes in the body, the most titillating being female genitalia. The preferred mode of gooey delivery in the accusers' frenzied minds was the broomstick; any sexual overtone was entirely intentional. It is unclear how old the idea was, but the first known mention is from the 1230s in a demonological tractate by Roland of Cremona, and the idea was enthusiastically adopted.

Scopolamine, present in mandrake (*Mandragora officinarum*) and henbane (*Hyoscyamus albus/niger*) may induce a sensation of flying and hallucinatory intoxication. High concentrations of hyoscyamine in deadly nightshade (*Atropa bella-donna*) may block out any sense of reality before sending the user into a deep sleep followed by amnesia. Other ingredients labelled as deliriant included datura, hemlock, opium poppy, soot and bats' blood, but even against that list, the suggestion by the philosopher Francis Bacon of "the fat of children digged out of their graves" frankly smacks of sensationalism. Sometimes monkshood (*Aconitum*) was also cited, not because it is a deliriant but because it contains aconitine, which lends a crawling sensation to the skin and the idea of growing fur or changing into an animal.

Australian musician and scholar Sarah Penicka has argued that flying ointment was "no more real than the concept of the Black Sabbath itself". She notes that the earliest recipes do not contain either henbane or mandrake, and that datura didn't even exist in Europe in the Middle Ages – and she has a point.

Once an idea is established, however, it is hard to quash, and the "hexing herbs" became firmly established in the popular imagination. They remain there today.

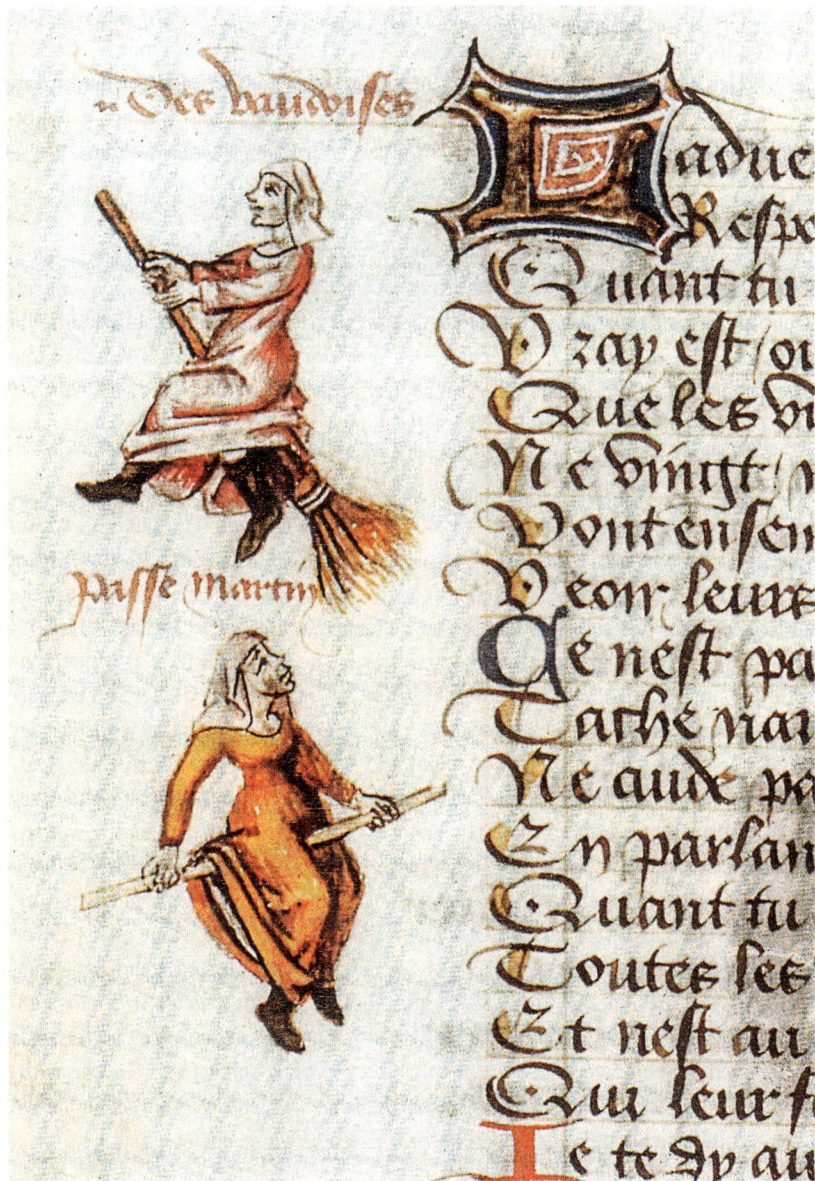

Above An illumination depicting two witches from
Martin Le Franc's *Le Champion des Dames*, is the first
known picture of flying witches in 1451.

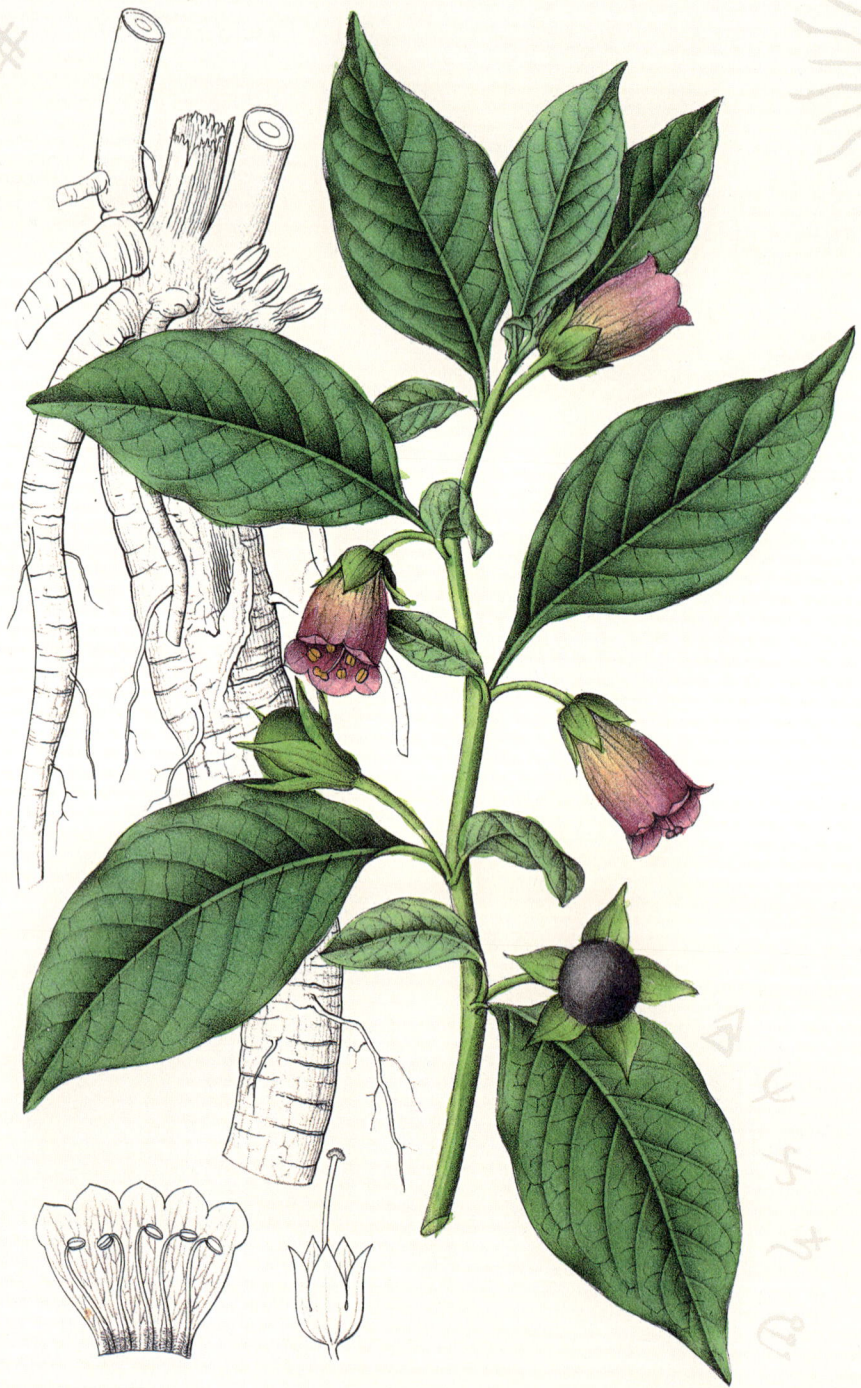

Deadly nightshade

Atropa bella-donna

Few in ancient Greece did not fear the Moirai, the three sisters who presided over the human lifespan. Clotho, "the spinner", spun the thread of life while Lachesis, "the apportioner" measured its length.

Atropos, "the inevitable", cut the thread. Perhaps it is fitting, then, that just two or three berries from the plant named for her, *Atropa bella-donna*, can kill a child.

Sometimes *Atropa bella-donna*'s deadly cocktail of toxins is ingested accidentally, perhaps by eating the flesh of a herbivore that has consumed the plant without ill effect. On other occasions it has been administered deliberately. It is rumoured the Roman emperor Augustus was poisoned by his wife Livia, who smeared juice from the "murderer's berry" onto some figs, and that deadly nightshade was one of the substances tested on condemned criminals by the Egyptian queen Cleopatra, searching for a suicidal potion that would not harm her beauty.

Cleopatra would not have used the plant's Latin name *bella-donna* ("beautiful lady"), but she may have been familiar with its use as a cosmetic to dilate the pupils. The practice was especially popular with Venetian women during the Renaissance.

Despite its obvious drawbacks, deadly nightshade has been a medicine cabinet staple since antiquity. Its traditional uses have ranged from alleviating teething pains and regulating heart palpitations and muscle spasms, to countering epilepsy and even use in surgery. Deadly nightshade has been suggested as a real-life candidate for the potion taken by Juliet, seeking to feign death. It can, as Shakespeare suggests, slow the heart rate and affect the nervous system, but only too often the effects may be permanent. Top of the real-plant suggestions for Romeo's draught, incidentally, is monkshood (*Aconitum*), from which there is no coming back.

Deadly nightshade is famous/notorious for one other attribute: as a deliriant hallucinogen. It was said in the Scottish Highlands that anyone using it would see ghosts. Phantoms may have been the least of their visions. Hyoscyamine and scopolamine figure highest in the herb's active ingredients. The herb can induce ecstatic and occasionally erotic hallucinations, alongside a dizzying range of side effects, from rapid heartbeat, seizures, blurred vision and confusion.

This has not stopped people using the dwale berry (from an old Scandinavian word for "trance") for millennia. It is said that the maenads (female followers) of Dionysus dilated their pupils with the herb before orgies, while the accusations against "witches" using deadly nightshade in fying ointment still echo into the twenty-first century.

Henbane

Hyoscyamus niger

In 1680 the world's worst neighbour, Mme Catherine Monvoisin, aka La Voisin, was executed in Paris for witchcraft and the deaths of around 1,000 people, though it is estimated she may have taken more than 2,500 lives.

Her favourite poison, in an armoury that included thornapple and arsenic, was henbane. Mme Voisin (whose name translates to "Mrs Neighbour") was only continuing a long tradition of grisly poisonings involving hyoscyamine, one of the major active compounds in henbane, which continued well into the twentieth century. The case of Dr Crippen, a seemingly mild-mannered homeopathist who killed his wife, smothered the body with quicklime and then absconded with his mistress, remains one of history's most infamous homicides. His radiotelegraphic arrest by "Marconigram" may have been up to the minute, but the murder weapon was positively antiquated.

Hyoscyamus is another member of the Solanaceae family, and there are several species, including *H. albus* (white henbane), *H. muticus* (Indian henbane) and *H. niger* (black henbane). Thanks to the alkaloids hyoscyamine and scopolamine, present in all three, they are a deadly crew. Black henbane is considered to contain the largest concentrations of toxins, and, in ancient Greek mythology, the souls of the dead wandering by the river Styx wore garlands of the herb as a warning to the living. Some say seers

at the Oracle of Apollo at Delphi used smoke from burning "Herba Apollinaris" to mimic the ravings of insanity, a useful tool in the prophecy business.

At the same time, physicians were discovering that henbane had its uses in medicine. The Ebers Papyrus, dating to c. 1550 BCE, is one of our best clues to ancient Egyptian herbal medicine. It suggests smoking Egyptian henbane as a sedative and painkiller, especially for toothache. The Roman physicians Dioscorides and Celsus also acknowledged its usefulness but did not care for its attendant dangers, so developed a safer, ointment form.

Ideas from antiquity filtered down the centuries, and the ancient Egyptian toothache wheeze was resurrected by quacks at medieval English fairs. Gullible sufferers were told their pain was due to worms eating their teeth and given a swill of henbane-laced mouthwash. When they spat it out, out came the "worms" – in reality, pieces of lute string. By the time the pain returned, the "doctor" had disappeared, but the patient may not have recalled the incident anyway, as henbane is also associated with memory loss. During the 1930s to '50s women giving birth were, much like their Roman forbears, given henbane – less, apparently,

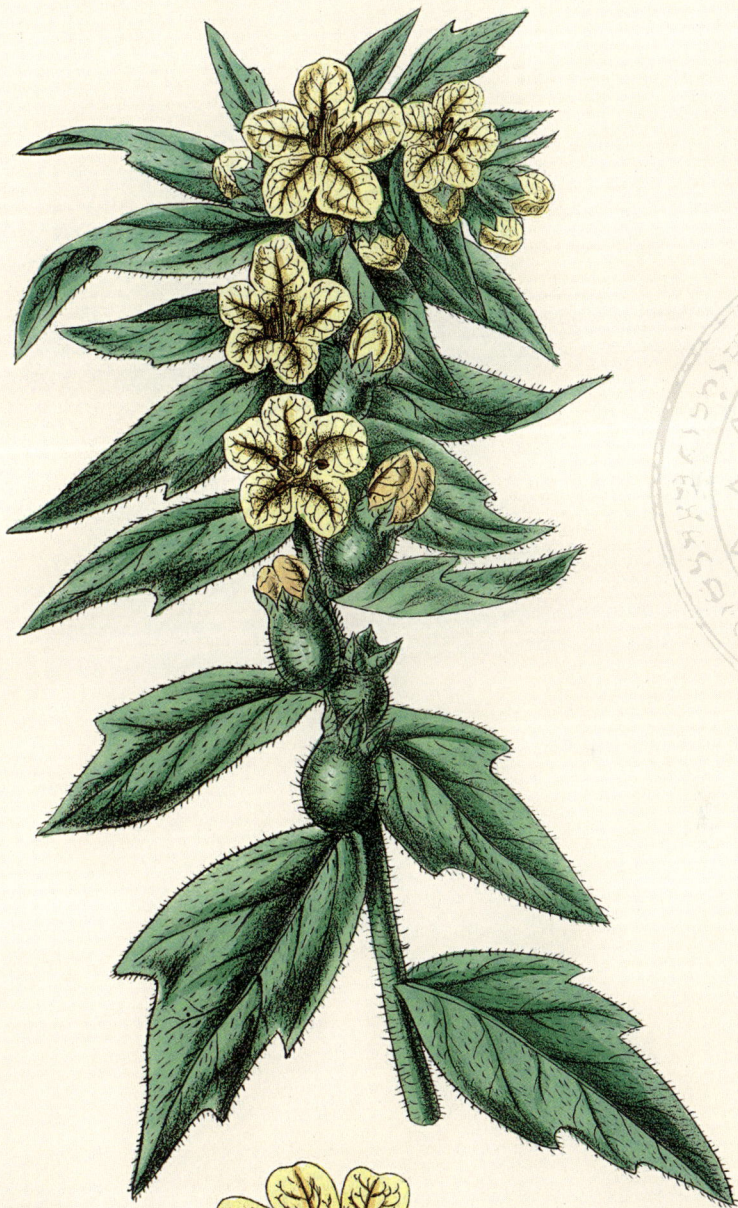

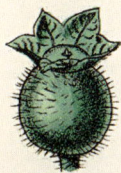

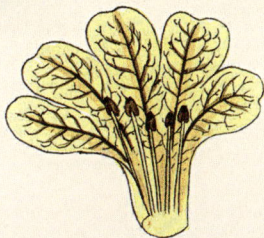

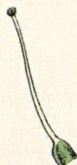

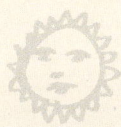

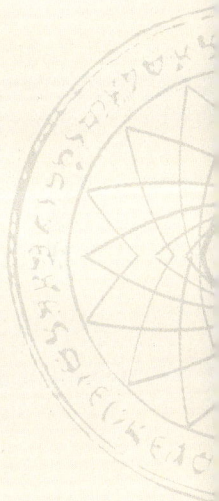

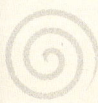

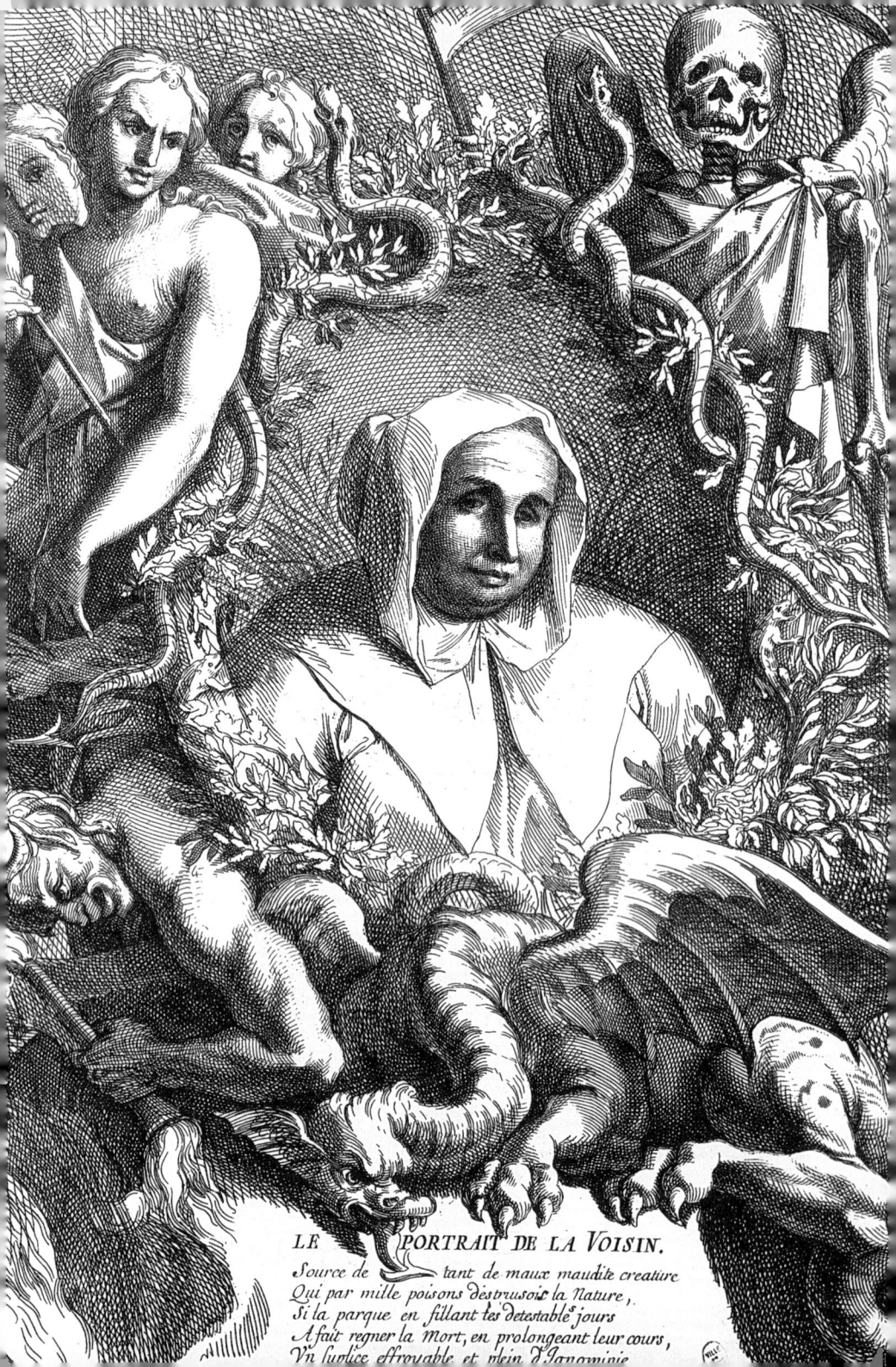

LE PORTRAIT DE LA VOISIN.

Source de   tant de maux maudite creature
Qui par mille poisons destruisoit la Nature,
Si la parque en fillant tes detestables jours
A fait regner la Mort, en prolongeant leur cours,
Vn supplice effroyable et plein d'Ignominie

for analgesic relief than for the opportunity to forget the pain afterwards.

The plant has sticky, hairy, jagged leaves and purple-veined, yellow-cream "eyes of the devil" flowers, and grows to around 1m (3ft) in height. It is easily recognized by an unpleasant odour, lending it the alternative name "stinking nightshade". Another name, "Jupiter's bean", is less easy to fathom.

Henbane acquired a seedy reputation in the Middle Ages and was denounced by the Church, especially Bishop Albertus Magnus, who reported that necromancers were using the herb to summon demons. It was even alleged it was being given to young people, rendering them suggestible enough to join Sabbat rituals. For the same reason the herb was sometimes used in love potions and, in the early twentieth century, was even investigated as an early truth serum. On the plus side, some said that people about to be tortured or executed were given henbane to help ease them into oblivion. A less bright idea from Germany was beer with *Hyoscyamus* seeds crushed into it for extra potency. Hyoscyamine and scopolamine dry out mucus membranes in the mouth, so drinkers also became thirstier with every stein they drank. The practice stopped with the 1516 Bavarian *Reinheitsgebot* (Purity Law) allowing only hops, barley and water in the brew, though yeast was later permitted.

From ancient times henbane's most famous use has been as a deliriant hallucinogen. Seeds, dried leaves or the crushed root are smoked or made into a tea which, depending on the dose, creates anything from a sense of drunkenness to powerful hallucinations. Users report pressure in the head, blurred or double vision, spasms in the jaw and neck, distorted senses of smell and/or taste, slurred speech and fits of aggression. An overdose can result in anything from vomiting, rapid heartbeat and palpitations to death. One of the most problematic aspects of taking the drug is that accurate dosage is extremely difficult to gauge. The levels of active compounds reflect not just the parts of the individual plant used, but also its quality, age and growing conditions – which is why a "lethal dose" has never been successfully quantified.

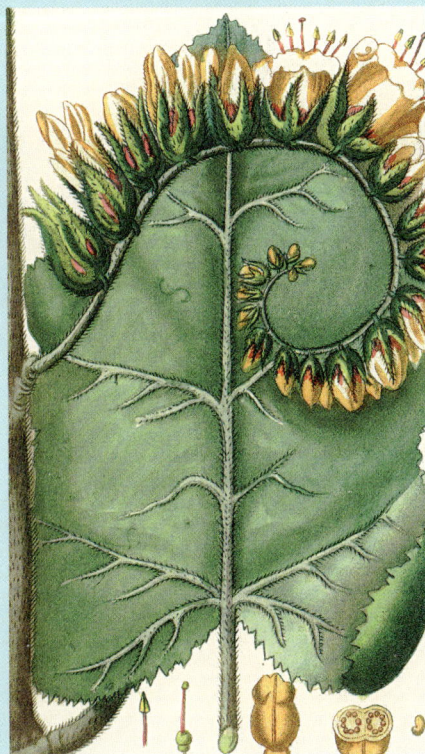

Above An illustration of *Hyoscyamus niger*.

Opposite Catherine Deshayes, known as La Voisin, was a fortune teller who traded love potions and poisons. She was burned at the stake in 1680 for being the alleged head of a ring of satanists.

Mandrake

Mandragora officinarum

There are few plants with more legends, folklore and superstition than the mandrake, the dangerous "apple of love" whose root looks like a tiny human – to those with a strong imagination...

Most ancient civilizations that spoke of the *Mandragora* (from "man" and "dragon") considered it a plant of the devil, possessing powerful magical properties. By the sixteenth century, mandrake roots that looked especially like humans (or fakes, including carved turnips and lumps of moulded earth) were sold as protective talismans and to aid fertility.

In a probable early attempt at demarcation by herb gatherers seeking to scare off competition, a long list of rules was created for gathering the plant, which was said to spring from the bodily juices of a hanged man. Finding the 30cm/12in-high rosette of leaves, with its pale green flowers and small, yellow fruits was hard enough, as it was said to be invisible during the day, though it shone like a star by night. The mandrake's long taproots were said to scream as they were pulled, causing madness or death. Only by stopping their ears, chanting the correct verses and performing certain rituals might someone gather the plants unscathed. The best method was to tie a dog to the plant, hide out of earshot, then call the mutt to retrieve the mandrake from the earth.

Mandragora does seem to have been worth the effort. In ancient Greece, it was popular in aphrodisiacs, thanks to its associations with Aphrodite, goddess of love, while the Romans used it to send patients into a drugged sleep before operations. It is thought mandrake was used in the "death wine" well-wishers gave to crucifixion victims to relieve them of their agonies on the cross. The condemned individual then slumped into a stupor, and soldiers cut them down for burial. Very occasionally, they might escape death altogether, but this was a high-risk strategy.

The Romans thought mandrake could cure madness or demonic possession, perhaps because of its properties as a narcotic and deliriant hallucinogen. Containing the usual alkaloids found in certain Solanaceae plants – atropine, hyoscyamine and scopolamine – it can affect the function of the nervous system in large doses, producing respiratory paralysis, coma and even death. Lower doses may induce pupil dilation, dizziness, drowsiness, dry mouth, nausea and delirium, including hallucinations and a "floating" sensation, which is why it was one of the classic ingredients of Flying Ointment. It is sometimes smoked or eaten, more usually drunk, either as a tea or soaked in wine, but largely avoided because of the nausea even low doses induce.

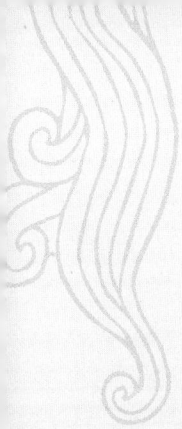

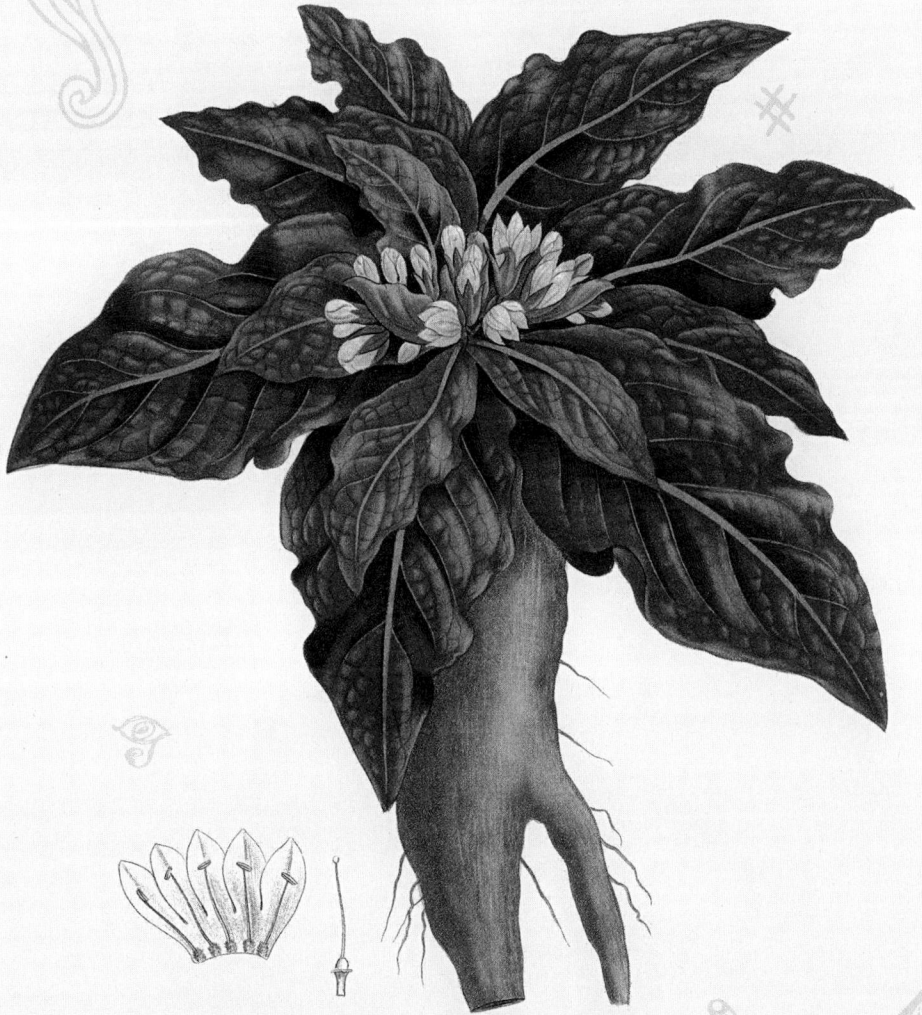

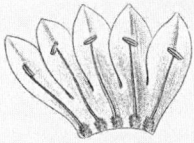

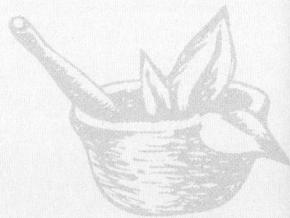

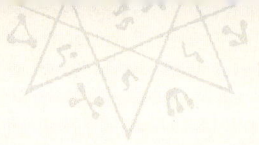

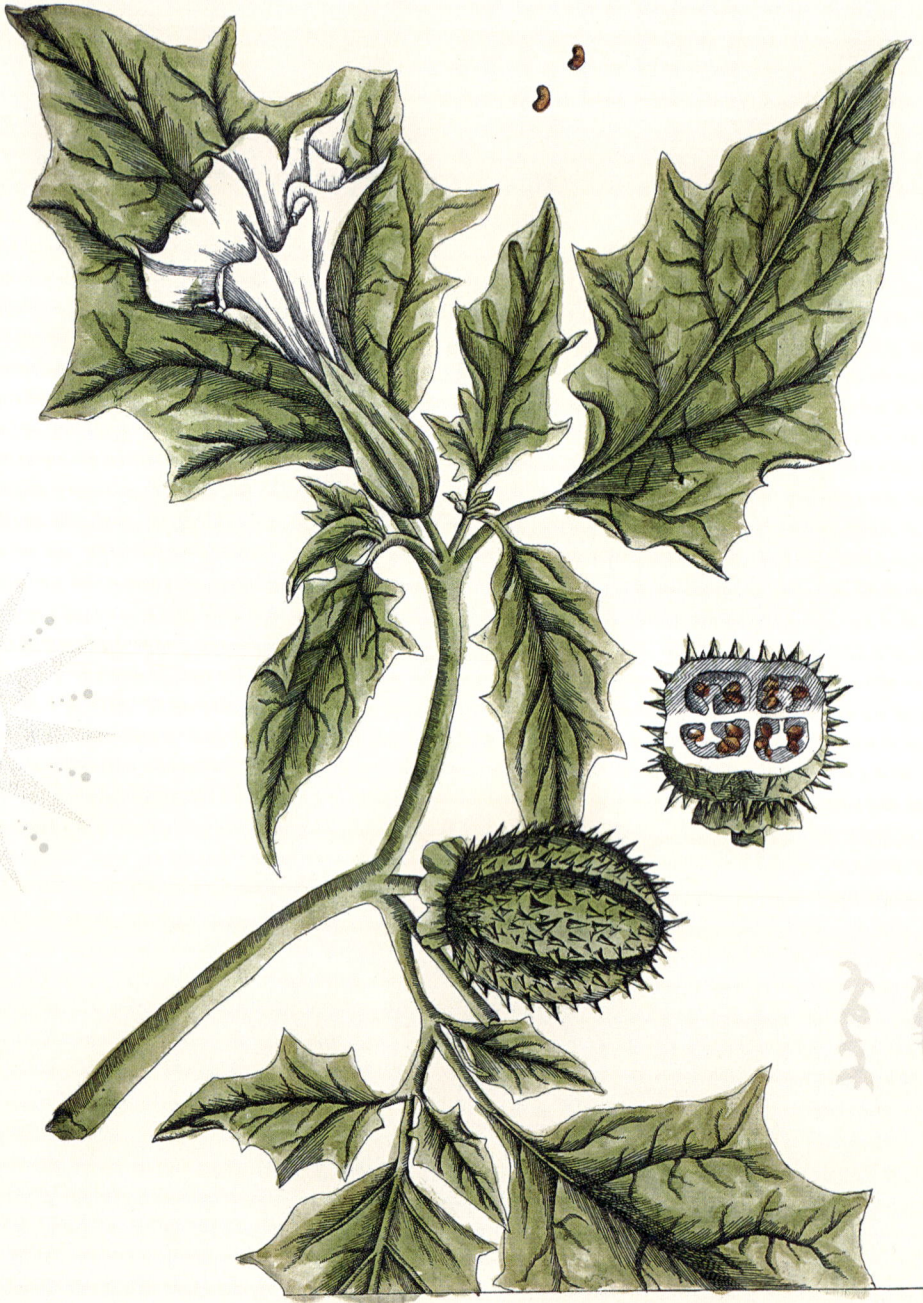

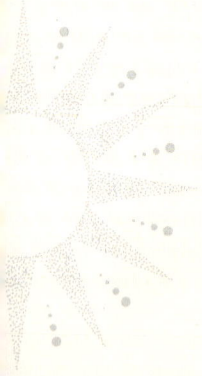

Thornapple

Datura stramonium

The artist Georgia O'Keeffe allegedly loved datura, her signature flower, for its delicate fragrance, reminding her of the cool of evening. Some might be surprised at this, as the plant is otherwise known for its foul odour.

Jimsonweed may stink, but for a few precious, night-time hours as it blooms, before fading at dawn, its perfume is intoxicating. So is the rest of the plant, if ingested. One of the most notorious deliriants, *Datura* is infamous for bad trips, filled with imagined terrors, distorted visions and horrifying auditory hallucinations. There are fourteen species of *Datura*, all with their own special demons. Every part of the "Devil's snare" is toxic, containing, like some of its cousins in the Solanaceae family, hyoscyamine and scopolamine.

There is a "thornapple" for almost every continent, easily recognized from softly jagged leaves and spiky fruit, and rites and rituals associated with the plant range across the world. In India it belongs to Shiva, the Destroyer, who is often depicted with *Datura* flowers woven into his hair. Offerings of the plant are often left for him or ritually burned. Less joyfully, it was given to widows expected to commit suttee – throw themselves on their husband's funeral pyre – as suggestibility is among the many effects of using the drug. The Muisca people of pre-Hispanic Colombia gave it to the wives of deceased chiefs before burying them alive; in Mexico, Aztec priests gave potential human sacrifices a *Datura*-based drink to produce a state of mental confusion.

In 1676, soldiers sent to suppress Bacon's Rebellion in Virginia ate a foraged salad and fell into a state of bizarre behaviour for 11 days before recovering and claiming to remember nothing. The rebellion started when the Governor of Jamestown refused to drive Native Americans from Virgina. Ironically, these were the very people who could have told him all about "Jamestown weed", later "jimsonweed", which was well-known across North America. Several indigenous communities in Virginia practised *huskanaw*, where young men were given nothing but datura for 18–20 days, during which they were mourned as if dead. If they survived the ordeal, they were said to have forgotten their childhood and were now ready for adult life.

Not for nothing does Raisa Sinclair, author of *A Field Guide to Deliriants*, declare the "Devil's weed" the "king of deliriants". Sinclair describes a particularly harrowing experience, starting with a very dry mouth and mental haze, followed by horrific hallucinations and distorted visions, then rising terror and a feeling of no control.

Angel's trumpet

Brugmansia

When writing their seminal *Plants of the Gods*, Richard Evans
Schultes, Albert Hofmann and Christian Rätsch were floored
by the beautiful plant known as angel's trumpets.

Yes, it was a plant of the gods, the authors eventually decided, but the gods can certainly be tricksy. For centuries, the *Brugmansia* group of plants was lumped in with *Datura* species, with which it shares many properties. The two genera have only relatively recently been specified, which makes separating their folklore difficult; stories are unclear and often interchangeable. One thing is certain: both are extremely dangerous. Horrific tales, from teenagers trying to chew off their own arms or rampaging through forests until there is no skin left on their feet, to the German lad who, in 2003, cut off his penis and tongue with garden shears and was left with no recollection of the incident afterwards, speak of the first, nearly always violent stage of *Brugmansia* intoxication. Many, however, fear more what follows: hallucinations and a coma, up to three days long. Some never wake.

This makes old reports even more terrifying. Giving dogs *Brugmansia* to enrage them for hunting sounds positively tame in contrast to a report from South America in the 1840s that seeds were added to Chicha beer to enable children to find gold deposits. It was even used to lace punishment drinks for naughty children, so the ancestors could scold them.

The Shuar community, who live mainly in Ecuadorian and Peruvian Amazonia, believe that real life is an illusion. Only by crossing to the spirit world can we understand and combat the forces of evil, via a person's *arutam* (soul). At puberty, or sometimes younger, boys undergo a ritual to acquire their first *arutam*, usually using ayahuasca to contact the spirits, who may appear in the form of jaguars or anacondas. In cases where this doesn't work, *Brugmansia* is employed. Once acquired, the *arutam* will last a few years before needing to be replaced.

Extreme care is needed when ingesting the plant. Even experienced shamans never take *Brugmansia* without an attendant, usually an apprentice, to care for them during each of the challenging stages. Individual plants have different levels of various alkaloids, including scopolamine and hyoscyamine, according to soil conditions, weather, altitude and damage. Shamans often grow their own personal plant, to more fully understand its effects.

Brugmansia is usually taken as a strong, unpleasant-tasting infusion made from the flowers or leaves; occasionally a stronger decoction is made

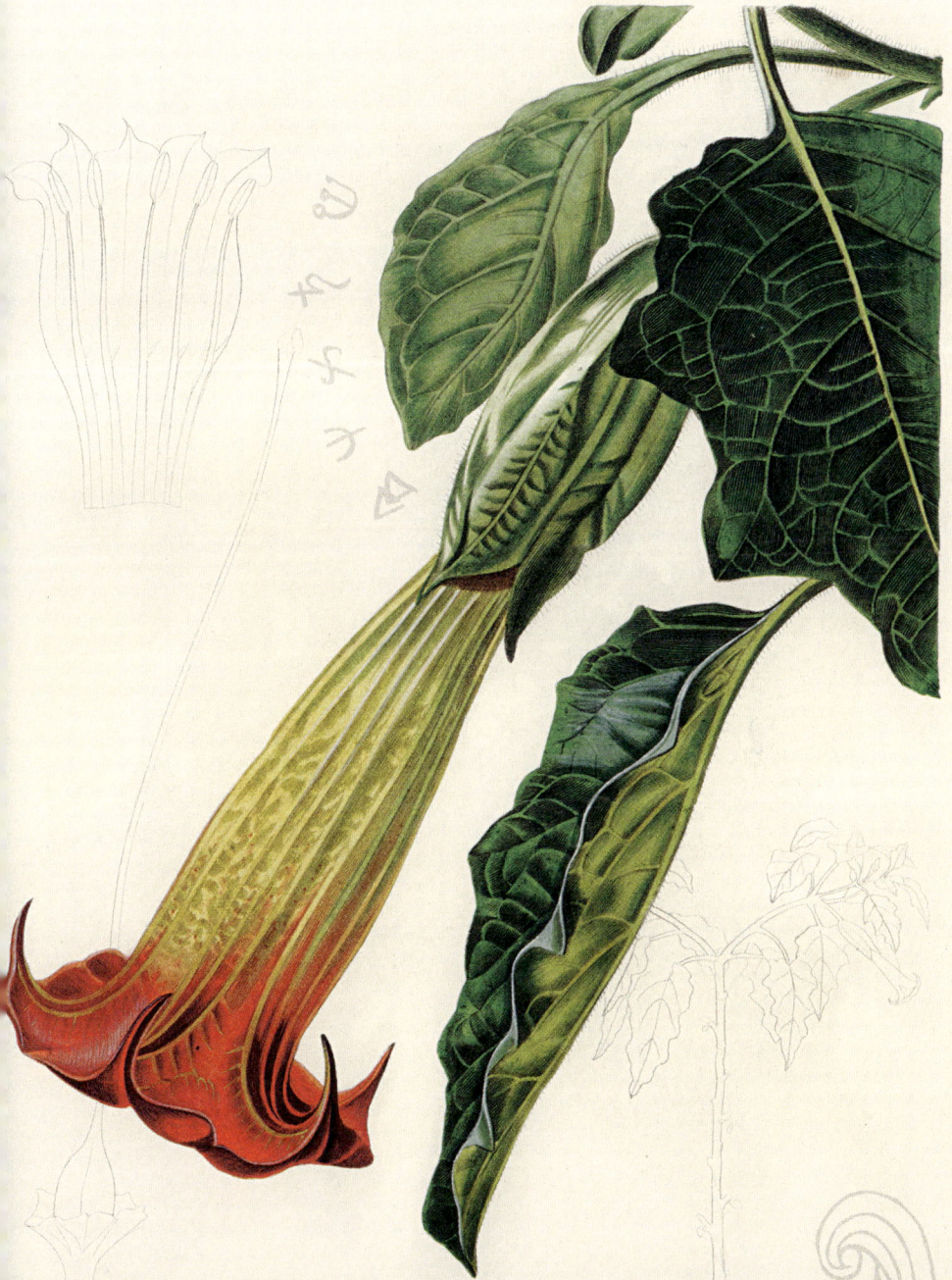

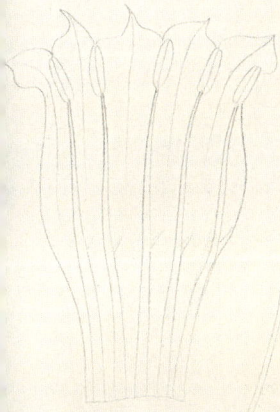

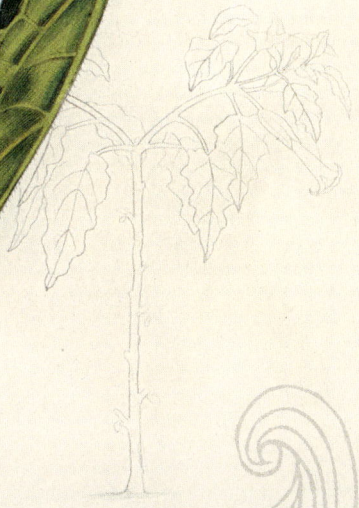

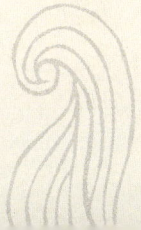

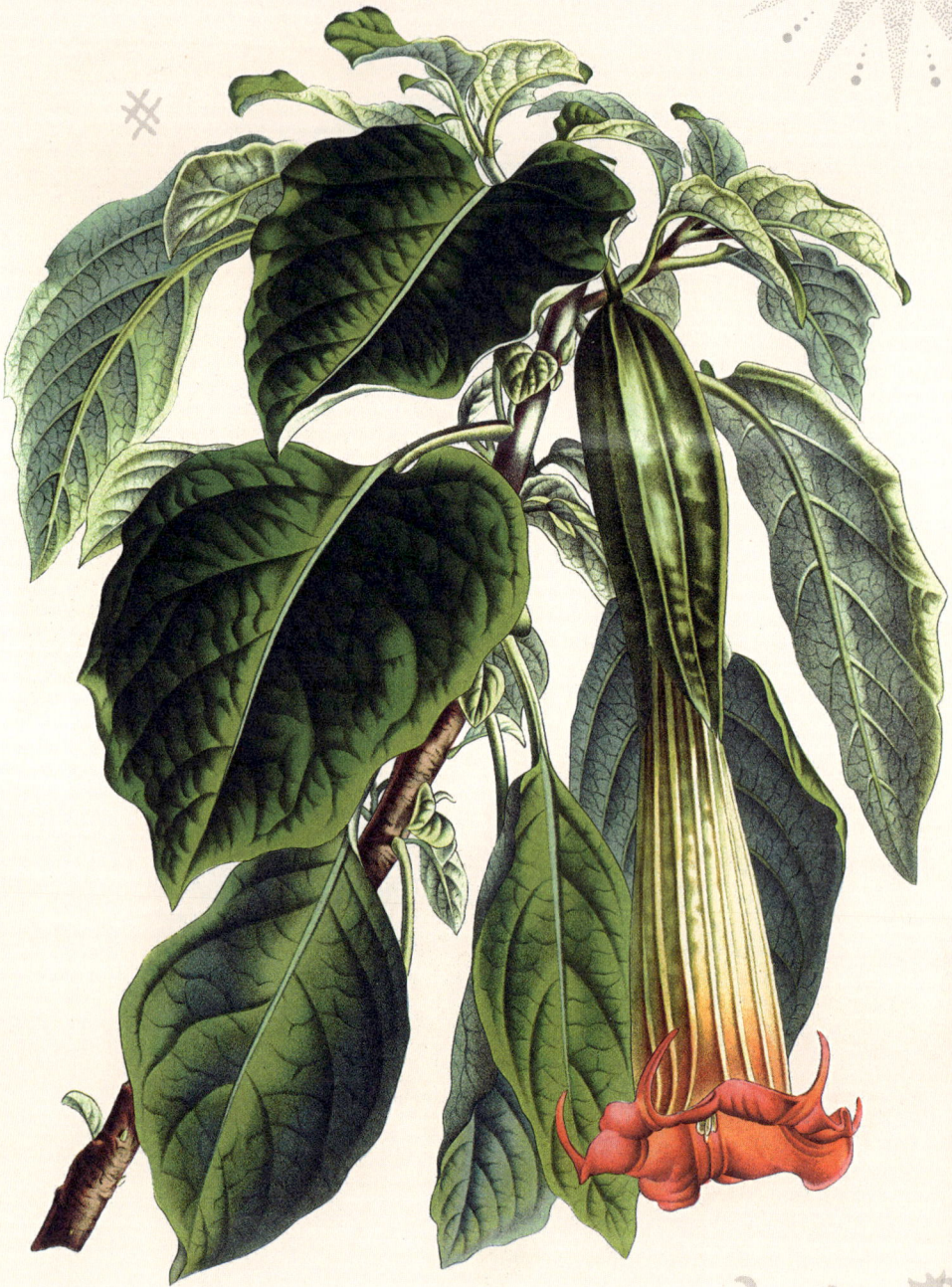

from bark scrapings. Very quickly an overwhelming fury rises in the user, which may include rolling eyes, foaming mouth, convulsions and visions. Many partakers feel capable of killing – and for a few, who have deliberately taken it to gain evil powers, this is enough. For Fernando Payaguaje, one of the last great shamans of the disappearing Secoya people, it was much harder – but vitally important – to remain stable, and to use *Brugmansia* to bring good via the next, difficult phase. The initial period of irrational fury, during which people often have to be restrained from harming themselves, is followed by several days of hallucinatory torpor, after which the subject may have been able to use it for divinatory or diagnostic purposes – or have little or no recollection of their experience.

Brugmansia's association with amnesia has been used for a range of unsavoury purposes, mainly, but not exclusively, in Colombia. Every year, the press reports on huge numbers of people who have been harmed or robbed after being rendered biddable by unknowingly ingesting "Devil's Breath". The US Overseas Security Council cites an unnamed source suggesting c. 50,000 victims, but it is hard to confirm exact figures. Such criminal activities were being written about by naturalist and explorer Alexander von Humboldt in the eighteenth century, however, and certainly still operate today.

For all its terrifying effects, this stunningly beautiful plant has its uses. In South America it is grown as protection against evil, placed at strategic points, such as steps, entrances, corners and at the edges of fields. If someone steals a part of the plant, any bad energy it has prevented goes with it – by contrast, when given freely as a gift, it brings magical protection. In Peru it is known as *Huaca*, or "plant of the tomb", grown in cemeteries and said to reveal graves that contain gold.

Brugmansia is also of great medicinal value to indigenous communities (usually applied externally, for obvious reasons).

Brugmansia is not a recreational drug, but there are still occasional poisonings, usually gardeners who accidentally ingest the plant, perhaps by accidentally touching it and then rubbing their face or eyes. Anyone who chooses to grow this staggeringly lovely plant should remember to wear gloves when tending it.

Peyote

*Lophophora
williamsii*

Tamatsi, the Blue Deer, is one of the most important deities
of the Huichol people, a bridge between gods and humans.
It is he who guides shamans through spiritual visions and
helps them find the sacred peyote.

The Huichol, also known as Wixárika, live mainly in Mexico and the southern United States. Tamatsi joins many other Huichol gods, creatures and plants, including Tayaupá, the Sun god; an eagle that links the sky and the Earth; and maize, the staff of life. During a peyote ceremony, a Huichol shaman may be said to transform themselves into a deer, via a *nierika* (door to the spirit world) revealing truths about both humans and the gods.

Peyote is a small, slow-growing, spineless cactus with long taproots, pink-white flowers and flattish, pumpkin-like shoots which, when harvested, are known as buttons. The plant contains more than 60 alkaloids, with one of the most powerful considered to be the entheogen mescaline. Manifesting in brightly coloured, kaleidoscopic visions, auditory hallucinations and variously altered senses of time and self, peyote has been used ritually and medicinally for, possibly, millennia.

According to Huichol legend, the first expedition to gather the sacred *peyotl* ("divine messenger" in Nahuatl, the Huichol language) was led by Tatewari, god of fire, who is often depicted with peyote in his hands or feet. Ever since, once a year, sometimes

biannually, pilgrims have undertaken the same journey across the sacred desert of Wirikuta to the mountains where the light is born. Usually travelling by car or bus these days, they complete the last part on foot, carrying gifts in baskets on their backs. As they near the mountains, after confession and purification, cleansing and prayer, they listen to a shaman's stories and chants and consume peyote, entering an imaginary Otherworld, firstly through the Gateway of the Clashing Clouds, and then the Opening of the Clouds.

At last, guided by the shaman, they begin their physical search, looking for the sacred deer tracks leading to the *hikuri* (peyote buttons). The shaman ritually "shoots" the first plant, and everyone makes offerings to it before filling their newly emptied baskets from surrounding cacti. They gather enough for themselves and a little to sell, but do not take the whole plant, ensuring there is enough left to resprout.

Peyote is important to the Huichol because ingesting it allows them to see the world from the cactus's point of view, but they are far from the plant's only enthusiasts. Many communities have their own rituals and Richard Evans Schultes, the

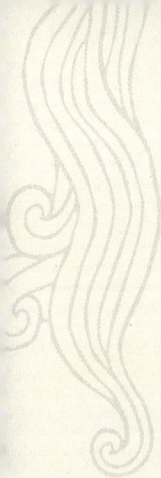

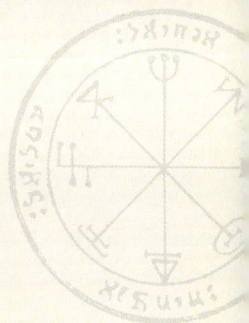

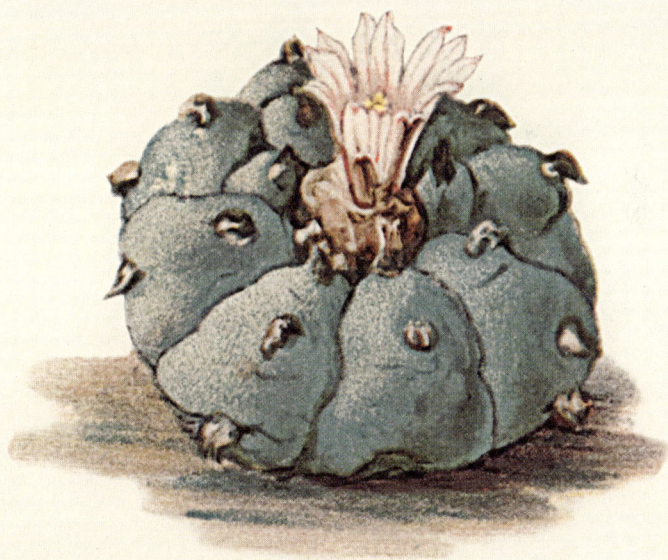

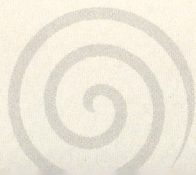

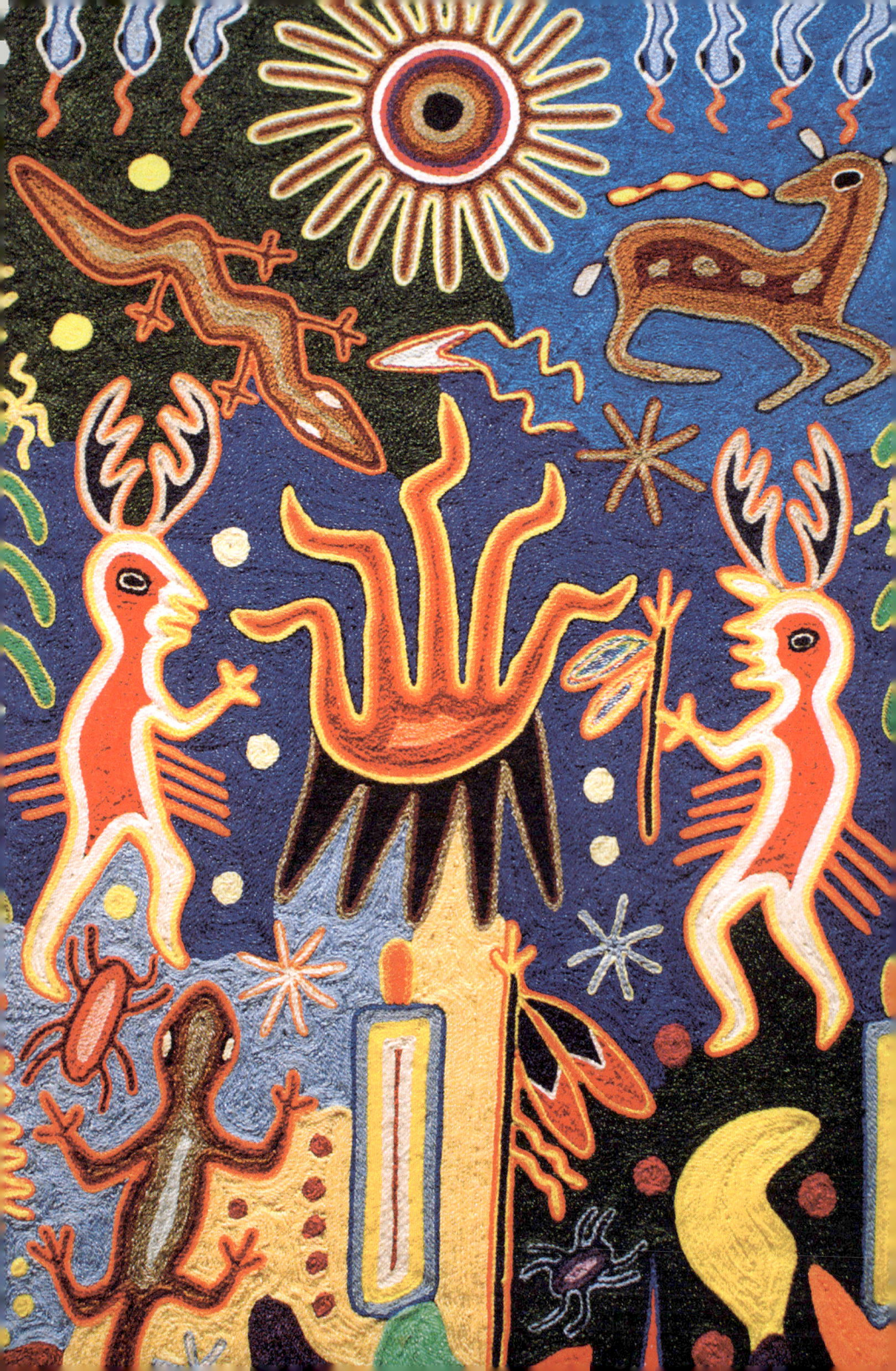

revered ethnobotanist, suggests that it was known among ancient peoples, including the nomadic Chichimeca, at least 1,890 years before the arrival of the Europeans. Recent archaeological remains containing peyote date back even further.

As usual, early modern Spanish missionaries were horrified by the ceremonies, but in their eagerness to denounce the "demonic" practices they have left us with colourful descriptions. Some, including large circles of men and women, all-night singing, dancing and music, sound not dissimilar to today's ceremonies.

Perhaps peyote's most widespread use is by an estimated 300,000 people from more than 40 US and Canadian First Nations, via the Native American Church. Founded around 1890 in Oklahoma territory and sometimes known as Peyotism or the Peyote Religion, the Church blends indigenous beliefs with elements from Christianity. Practices, including the means of consumption, differ wildly, but a few elements are central, including the reverence of a Great Spirit, and the use of peyote, often alongside tobacco.

Mescaline was one of the first alkaloids to be scientifically isolated, in 1897, by German pharmacologist Arthur Heffter, allowing for its synthesis in 1919 by an Austrian chemist, Ernst Späth. It became an influential substance for beat writers including William S. Burroughs, Jack Kerouac and Allen Ginsberg, who were often inspired by Aldous Huxley's descriptions of taking mescaline in his autobiographical work *The Doors of Perception* (1954).

A bitter substance, whether eaten or brewed as a tea, peyote may induce dizziness, headaches, nausea, vomiting and diarrhoea as well as the more famous hallucinations and clarity of thought. It is illegal in many countries, though rarely banned as an ornamental plant. There is an exception in US law: thanks to the American Indian Religious Freedom Act Amendments of 1994, any member of the Native American Church may ingest the cactus as part of a religious sacrament. In Mexico, despite the substance being illegal, there is a thriving "peyote pilgrimage" tourist industry.

Peyote is an increasingly endangered species. This is not due to its use as an entheogen, or to the few remaining *peyoteros*, who have always harvested the buttons sustainably. Strip-gathering by poachers and cattle farming is adding to the plant's vulnerability in the United States and, while legally protected in Mexico, its habitat is threatened by silver mining. Cultivation is possible but slow; it takes 13 or more years for a plant to mature.

Opposite A traditional Huichol yarn painting from the National Museum of Anthropology in Mexico City.

San Pedro

Trichocereus macrogonus
var. *pachanoi*

Like its namesake Saint Peter, *Trichocereus macrogonus* var. *pachanoi* is said to hold the keys to heaven, though the Spanish missionaries who brought the saints to South America would not have enjoyed the comparison.

The indigenous people the missionaries came to convert in South America were forced to hold their ceremonies in secret; even today, healing rituals involving *huachuma* (San Pedro cactus) are held by night.

San Pedro itself enjoys the night-time, bursting into enormous, fragrant flowers to attract hummingbirds and moths. Some say ingesting *huachuma* causes a participant's subconscious to "bloom" in a similar way.

The cactus, whose spiny columns can rise as high as 4m (13ft), is sometimes mistakenly assumed to be several plants growing together. Each branch has distinctive "ribs" to add rigidity and store water. A typical plant has seven ribs and may eventually sport ten or more. It is believed that the most spiritually powerful specimens have just four, representing the four winds. A major "teacher plant", *huachuma* is one of the most important ingredients in a shaman's medicine chest across Peru, Bolivia and Ecuador, and the main constituent of *cimora*, a traditional brew containing other hallucinogenic plants.

Reverence for San Pedro dates back millennia. In the Stela of the Cactus Bearer, a monolith from the Chavin civilization of Northern Peru, a *huachumero* (a shaman working with *huachuma*) is depicted holding the cactus. It appears there were originally four such stele, dating to around 750 BCE.

A modern shaman includes San Pedro with other sacred objects on *mesas* (altars) for use in healing. San Pedro is easily purchased from local markets, but the shaman may have their own store; the longer it is kept, the stronger the mescaline content. The cactus is boiled for many hours, strained and cooled for drinking at midnight. It is generally considered to bring a less stimulating but more stable experience than peyote.

Depending on the strength of the brew, effects may include dreamlike (sometimes nightmarish) visions and hallucinations; it is used to diagnose illness, purify evil and receive guidance from the ancestors. *Huachuma* is sometimes known as an *abuelo* (or grandfather) medicine and traditionally grown close to the home, protecting the family and allowing everyone to live peacefully together.

Even the missionaries had to admit San Pedro was a useful medicinal plant. Research has revealed anti-inflammatory and possible antibiotic properties, and there has been interest in its potential use to reduce blood pressure and nervous tension.

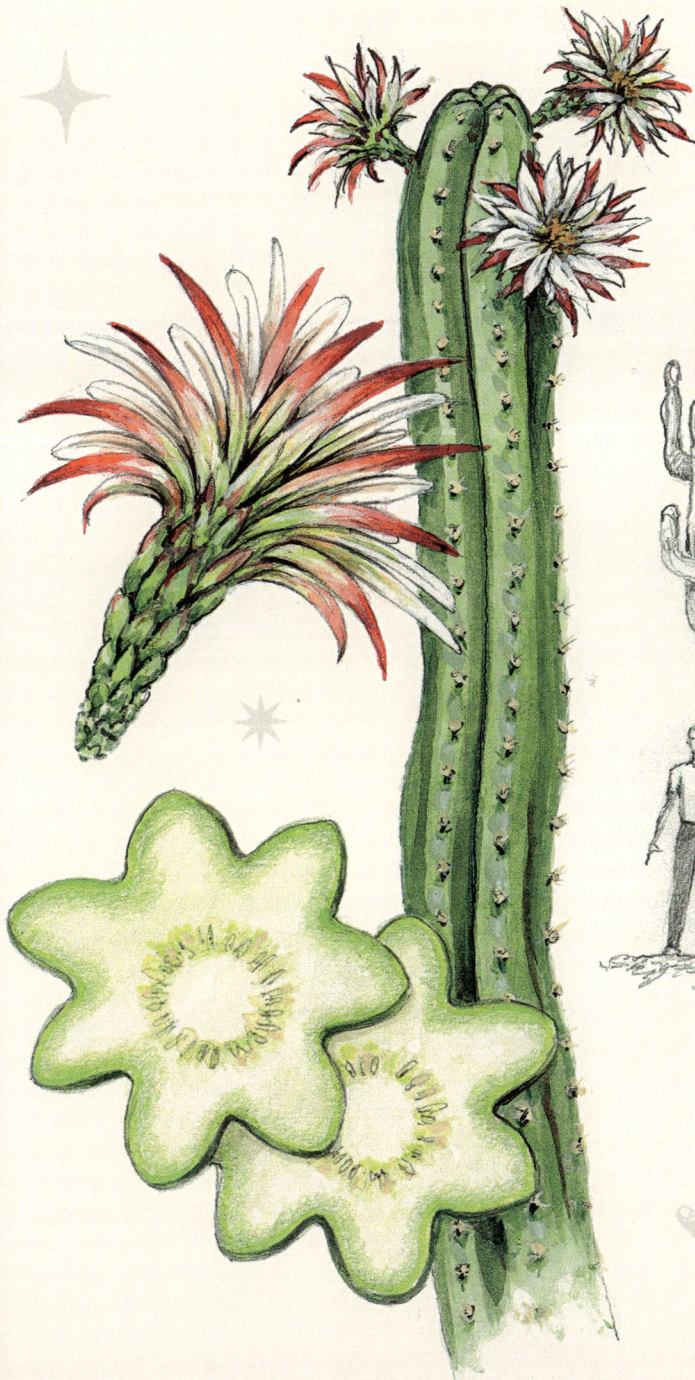

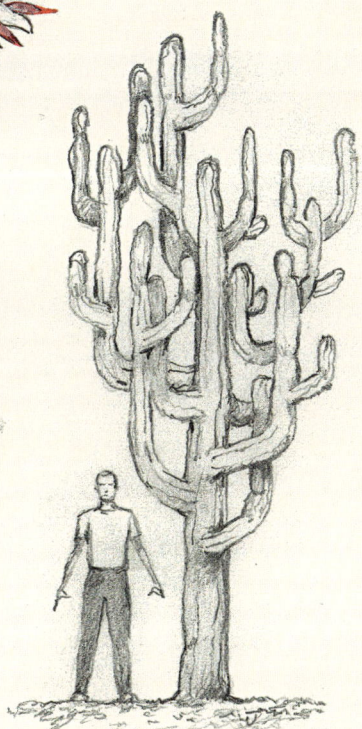

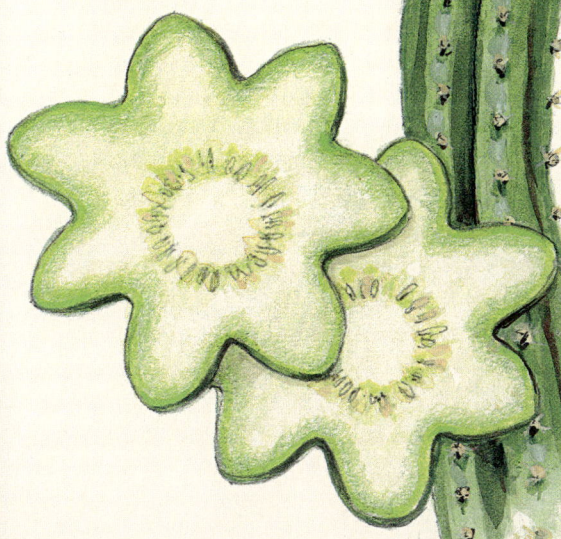

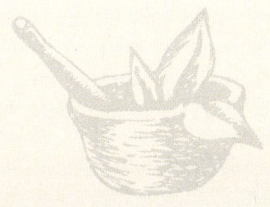

War on Drugs

The horrors of war are too much for most people to
contemplate, not least for the soldiers who have to fight in
them. It is hardly surprising that few battles have been fought
without a little help from one substance or another.

The most obvious is alcohol. The ancient
Greek warriors of Homer's *Iliad* drink wine
for fortification, solace and camaraderie; it
is even thrown onto the fire as libation to the gods.
Soldiers have done much the same ever since.
The Russians drank vodka; the Germans, beer; in
America, it was mainly whiskey. Until 1970 British
sailors enjoyed a daily ration of navy-strength rum,
its extremely high proof not there for the rufty-tufty
tars but to ensure that if the barrels were accidentally
smashed, soaking the gunpowder stored next to
them, it would still ignite.

Stimulants keep combatants alert and imbue an
enhanced sense of bravado. Inca warriors chewed
coca leaves. Some say Viking Berserkers found their
legendary crazed courage and oblivion to pain from
Amanita muscaria mushrooms (see p. 131). Modern
scholars are less sure – though only the substance
is disputed, not the suggestion that "something"
was ingested. Top of the scary list is currently
Hyoscyamus niger, black henbane (see p. 168).

Drugs may also be used as instruments of
warfare. Hannibal pretended to retreat from a
besieged city after spiking its wine with mandrake.
As soon as the insurgents were drugged, his men
returned with a vengeance – and falcata swords.

Substances relieve two of the worst aspects of
warfare: pain and depression; and one of the most

insidious: boredom. Morphine did the trick during the
American Civil War. It has been with us ever since;
cocaine is another omnipresence. During the First
World War Harrods department store was just one
outlet selling cigarette case-style kits containing
morphine, cocaine, syringes and spare needles for
young women to send to their sweethearts in the
trenches. Things became complicated in 1916 when
a national panic about the evils of cocaine restricted
dispensation to official prescription, often under
the brand name "Forced March". The Second World
War saw the rise of synthesized substances. Nazi
troops and Japanese kamikaze pilots were given
the methamphetamine Pervitin. Allied troops took
similar drugs, just with different names.

The Vietnam War coincided with the psychedelic
explosion back home. An estimated 50% of
American soldiers used some kind of drug, perhaps
amphetamine or other psychedelic, perhaps
marijuana, but also heroin and cocaine. In later years
the percentage rose to circa 70%.

From Troy to the Somme, the Gulf to Afghanistan,
no conflict is drug-free. Could any of us do the things
required of a soldier in wartime without a little
numbing around the edges?

Opposite It's believed that half of American soldiers
in the Vietnam war used some kind of drug. This
illustration shows a stoned American GI smoking pot.

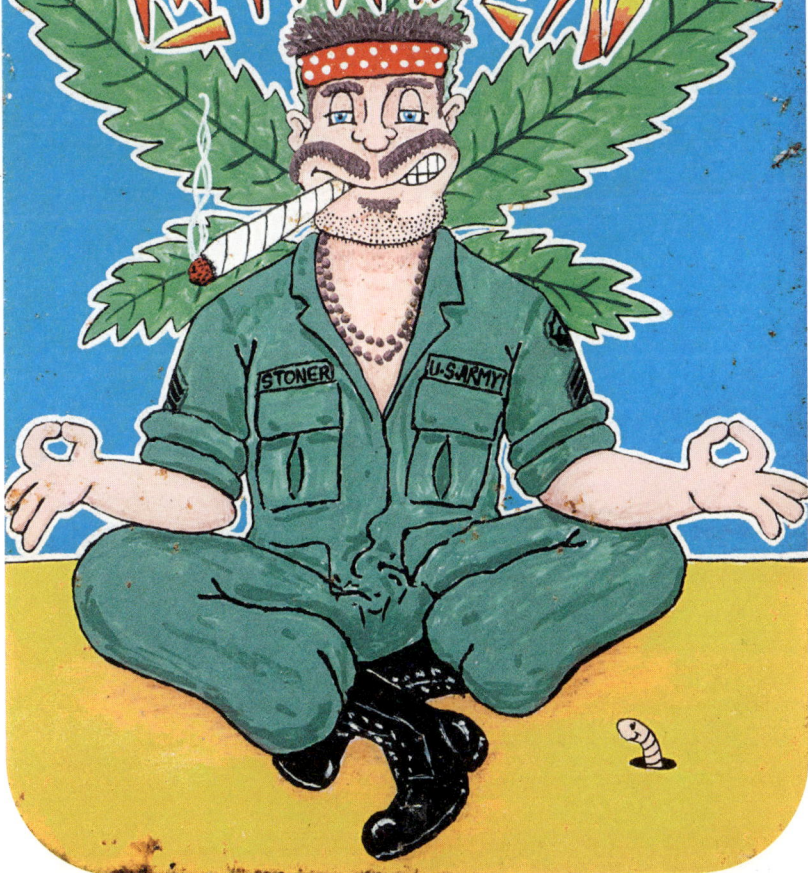

Chapter 10:
The Psychotropic Medicine Chest

Mind-altering drugs have a long medicinally oriented history. Some, such as ayahuasca, peyote and psilocybin, are specifically entheogenic, leading users through spiritual journeys to find answers, often to health problems, both physical and emotional. Other psychotropic drugs, while still working with the mind, do not necessarily involve vision quests or conjure hallucinations, instead engaging in other ways to enhance mood or otherwise retain a healthy mind.

St John's wort

(Hypericum perforatum)

The summer solstice and midsummer, the longest day of the year, arrive slightly apart from one another. The former usually falls around 21 June; the latter on 24 June, a day that is sacred to St John the Baptist.

Any plant that reaches its zenith at the turn of the year has always been considered magical. The golden-flowered St John's wort, whose many names also include penny John, rosin rose and touch-and-heal, is considered one of the most protective of those midsummer plants. A symbol of the Sun, it was especially useful on St John's Eve, 23 June, when spirits and witches were abroad. It was sometimes burned; people might jump through the incense-like smoke. Sprigs were hung from doorways in homes and cattle sheds or worn as protective charms against the evil eye.

The ancient Greeks gave the name *hypericum* (from *hyper* – "above" – and *eikon* – "apparition") to a protective herb they hung over statues; whether they were referring to today's plant is unclear. *Perforatum* refers to the translucent glands in hypericum's leaves, which look like holes.

St John's wort was used in divination games, perhaps to find a girl's chances of marrying or, less enjoyably, someone's life expectancy. The devout might sleep with a sprig under their pillow to dream of the saint and receive his blessing. The associations with St John continue until 29 August, traditionally the anniversary of his death by beheading, when dark splotches of "blood" appear on the herb's leaves. Red oil crushed from them was called "witch's blood", and rumoured to make a fine love potion.

St John's wort has been used in medicine for centuries, Nicholas Culpeper suggesting it boiled in wine for a range of ailments. From the mid-1990s medical research into claims for *Hypericum perforatum* as a potential treatment for mild and even severe depression, without the attendant side effects of synthetic antidepressants, seemed to produce encouraging results. The theory was that the herb's combination of phytochemicals, including hyperforin, work together to increase the activity of brain chemicals such as serotonin, helping to regulate mood.

New research has since added nuance to those early results and scientists now regard St John's wort with a more circumspect eye, noting its effects may be limited and there have been concerns it may increase symptoms of psychosis in some. There is also evidence that *Hypericum perforatum* can influence how certain other drugs are broken down in the body, including the contraceptive pill. Anyone considering St John's wort should treat it like any other drug and consider carefully any possible contraindications.

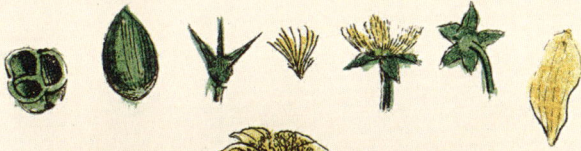

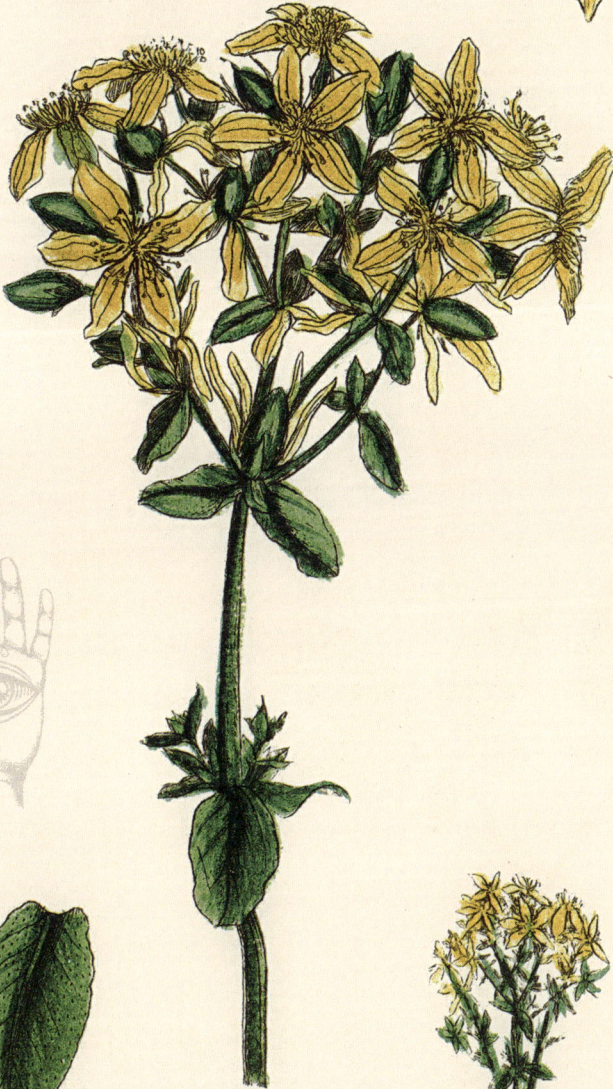

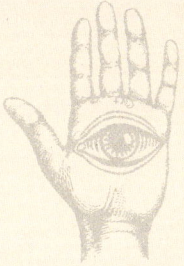

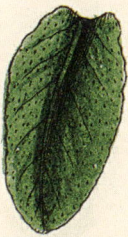

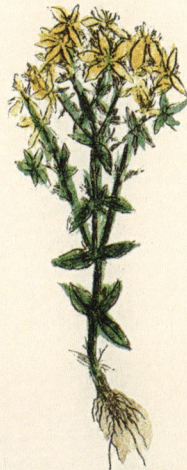

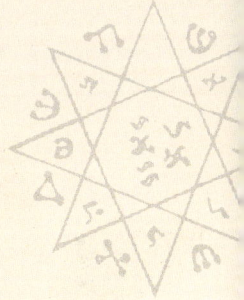

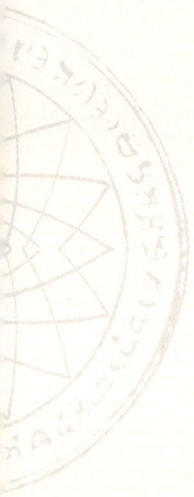

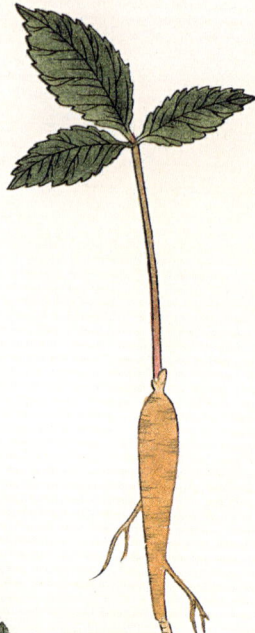

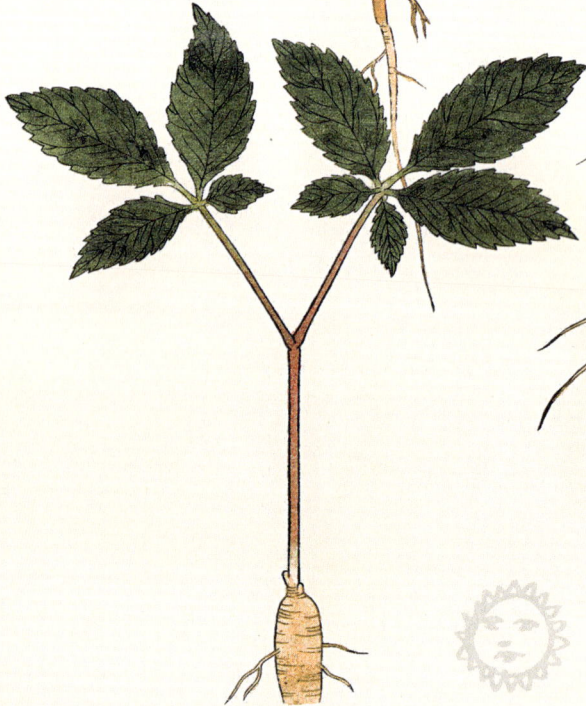

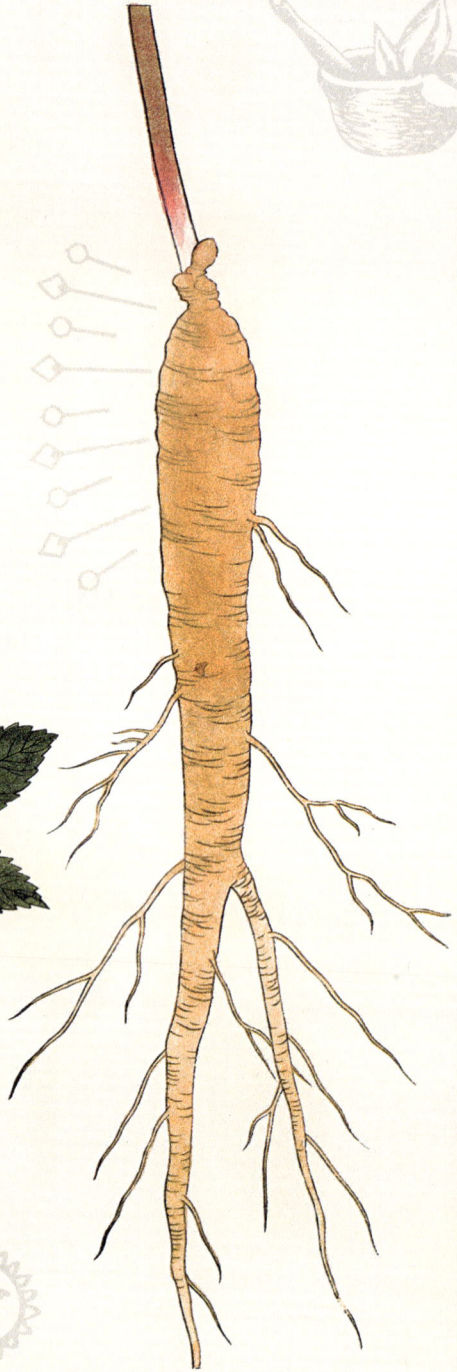

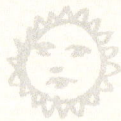

Ginseng

Panax ginseng

Many centuries ago, a schoolboy went to the caves of
Gwaneum at Mount Jinak, South Korea, to pray for his sick
mother. In a dream, the mountain's guardian spirit sent the
boy to find a magical, cure-all plant with red fruits.

Wild ginseng is at the heart of Korean ancestor worship, connected to mountain gods and crows, the bird of filial piety. The three-legged crow Samjok-o, who lives in the sun, is particularly associated with ginseng, but the "king of herbs" has been revered across the Far East for at least 5,000 years, bringing with it all manner of deities, legends and origin myths. One Chinese story sees a fairy banished from heaven for bathing in a sacred lake, marrying a mortal and then bequeathing ginseng to cure the ills sent by the heavenly father as punishment, while as far back as the sixth century Taoist priests were writing of necromancers using ginseng with cannabis to scry into the future.

The name *Panax* comes from the Greek *pan* (all) and *akos* (cure). *Panax ginseng* is loved as an antioxidant-rich tonic for dozens of ailments and is popular for its reputed neuroprotective properties. The practitioners of both Indian Ayurvedic and traditional Chinese medicine (TCM) use it as a matter of course. While neither a hallucinogenic or classically mind-altering substance, ginseng is anecdotally believed to improve stress-related conditions and

memory loss – claims that are increasingly being investigated on a more scientific basis. In America, a close cousin, *Panax quinquefolius*, has been equally prized as a "universal" medicine, initially by First Nations communities, then by practically everyone, leaving the wild plant severely endangered. It is vanishingly rare in Asian countries too, but thankfully has been cultivated since around 11 BCE.

Like the (unrelated) mandrake (see p. 172), the root often resembles a small human, leading to similar superstitions. Unlike *Mandragora officinarum*, however, ginseng will not scream as it is pulled, leading to instant madness, but intricate superstitions still cling to its harvesting. On finding a ginseng shoot, shout: "Stick!" to freeze it and prevent escape. The head of the hunting party will call: "What variety?" and, according to the number of leaves and shoots, indicating the plant's age, the finder will reply with a specific code word. Six offshoots suggest a very old and precious specimen.

Only the party leader may dig a ginseng root, covering it first with a straw hat before tying it up so the "little man" cannot run away.

Catnip

Nepeta cataria

Not all cats react to nepetalactone, the main active compound in catnip, but those that do are unforgettable. One whiff and a previously sleepy kitty explodes into a crazy 10 minutes of rolling, purring, rubbing, mewing hyperactivity.

Obviously, scientists cannot ask their subjects what the experience is like, but it may be psychedelic, similar to the hallucinogen LSD. A *Nepeta* high will last around 10 minutes, after which it will take around two hours for the moggy to "come down" and show interest again. Cats are among a group of animals with an extra sensory organ in the roof of their mouths. The vomeronasal gland channels chemicals to the brain, including pheromones from potential enemies – and mates. Catnip mimics female sex hormones, stimulating felines of both genders, though a few can become aggressive.

Native to Europe, Southwestern and Central Asia, catnip (also catmint and catwort) is one of more than 200 genera in the mint (Lamiaceae) family, some of which also contain nepetalactone in lesser quantities. The name *Nepeta* may derive from the ancient Roman town Nepete (modern-day Nepi) where the herb was either cultivated or grew freely. Cataria is from the Latin *cattus*. Traditionally a plant of Venus, the herb is usually associated with female gods, including the ancient Egyptian feline deities Bast and Sekhmet, the Norse goddess Freya, and the Celtic Cerridwen.

Nepeta cataria was a staple of medieval monastery herb gardens, taken for fevers and colds, colic, gastric problems, rheumatic swellings, and as a relaxant. Nicholas Culpeper recommended women seeking to conceive should take a catmint-infused bath, and it has been used in fertility charms and for menstrual cramps, though the herb is not recommended for pregnant women. *Nepeta cataria* is prepared by herbal practitioners as a traditional remedy for respiratory complaints, catarrh and sore throats and applied topically for minor wounds and skin problems. Humans sometimes smoke the dried catnip leaves with tobacco as a reputed sedative and (*very*) mild hallucinogen, while an infusion of catnip is thought to ease insomnia and anxiety – although it is advised that it should only be taken in small doses, and side effects include headaches and vomiting.

For susceptible kitties, eating rather than smelling catnip leaves – unusually, fresh leaves are more potent than dried – results in a distinct chilling-out. This has been observed in big cats too. Kittens do not develop the sensory trait until about three months old. Overdoses are rare, but eating too many leaves can cause sickness. Eating catnip root, however, can cause aggression in felines and humans alike.

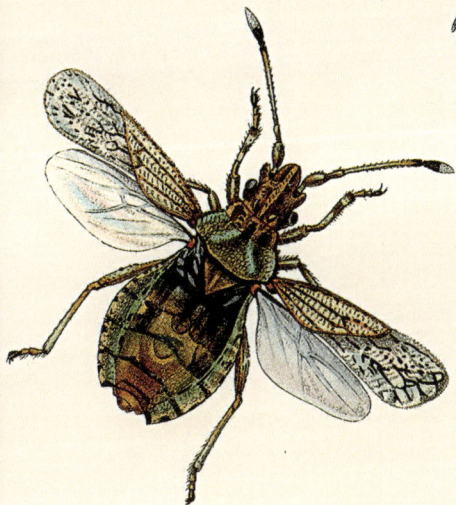

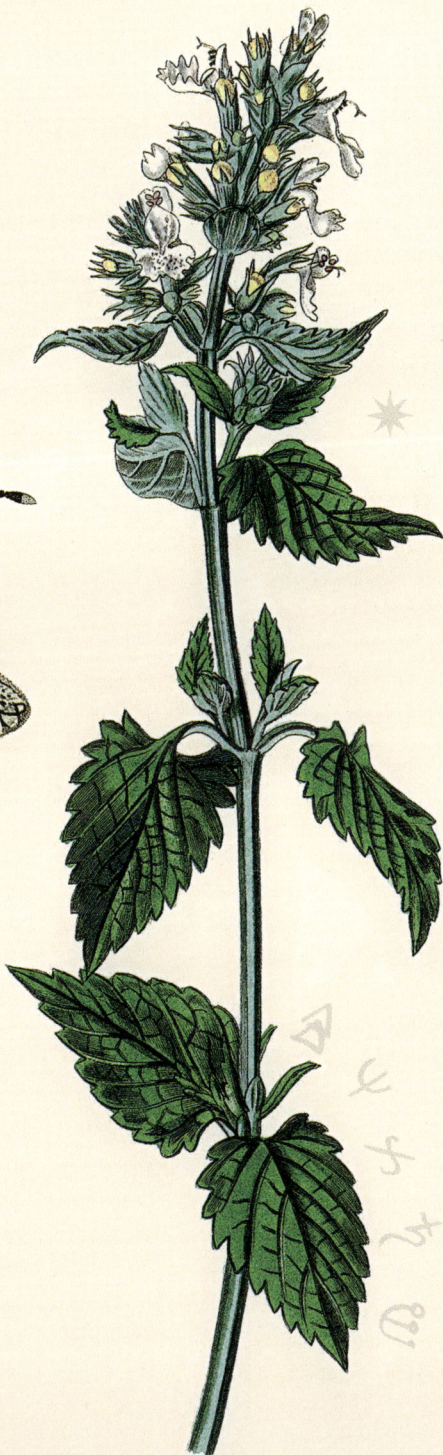

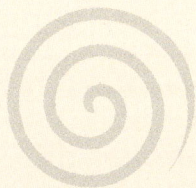

Drugs of the Future

In *Magic Medicine*, Cody Johnson points out that even today many of us still subscribe to the old idea of psychedelic substances epitomizing a spaced-out, 1960s danger zone, well deserving of their generally illegal status.

A growing number of scientists are now, however, prepared to take a second, clinically controlled look at hallucinogens, including revisiting research that faltered long ago. Such work may have become legally hog-tied during the non-discriminative War on Drugs or have involved unorthodox practices later discredited. In a world terrified by the very mention of "drugs" it has taken courage to suggest that however wacky the methodologies, there may have been something in them.

Work has restarted, for example, examining the almost unique properties of *Tabernanthe iboga* in countries that have not banned the drug. Modern trials exploring theories proposed by Howard Lotsof back in 1962 (see p.28) tentatively suggest that ibogaine appears to affect the brain's frontal cortex, effectively rewiring previous memories of addiction, though the process is not without very real dangers, especially if the body isn't "told" about the brain's neurological overhaul.

More often psychedelic substances are being investigated as aids to psychotherapy. Unlike hard drugs such as heroin and cocaine, psychedelics are rarely addictive, not least because the experience can be unpleasant. In 2006 Dr Roland Griffiths at John Hopkins University revisited the ideas behind the Marsh Chapel Experiment (see p. 123) with largely similar results. Such work with psilocybin sparked renewed interest across the world. London's Imperial Centre for Psychedelic Research uses a range of imaging techniques to explore the brain's reaction to, and possible benefits of, magic mushrooms as a therapeutic aid for conditions as wide-ranging as severe depression, anorexia, chronic pain, post traumatic stress disorder, end-of-life anxiety and obsessive-compulsive disorder.

Some of the loudest buzz is around research about how two compounds within *Cannabis sativa* interact with our bodies' cannabinoid and other receptors. These compounds are tetrahydrocannabinol (THC) and cannabidiol (CBD). THC and CBD are chemically similar, but not identical, so interact with cannabinoid and other receptors in different ways, explaining their different effects. THC is largely responsible for marijuana's "high", whereas CBD produces different effects on the nervous system, so has been of interest for therapeutic applications, such as to help with social anxiety and chronic pain.

Perhaps it is about time Big Pharma began to rethink previously shunned substances. Many conventional drugs currently on the market have their own problems and the twenty-first century faces, possibly, the biggest mental health crisis humanity has known. Nothing can afford to be off

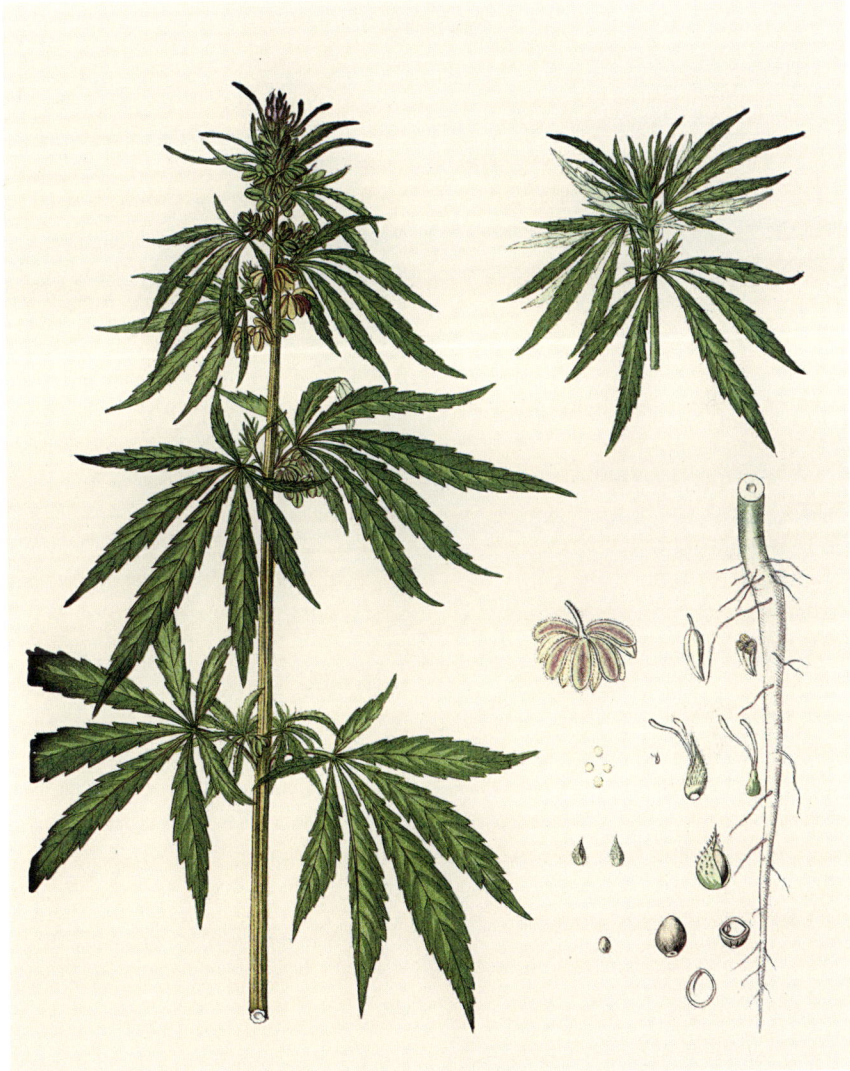

the table, and psychoactive plants, from ayahuasca to peyote, may have a role to play yet. Maybe the moment has come to put prejudice behind us and start listening to what shamans have been telling us for a very long time.

Above *Cannabis sativa* is one of many plants being investigated for it's medicinal benefits today.

Glossary

Alkaloid – an organic compound containing nitrogen in the chemical structure; alkaloids often have physiological effects on the human body

Aphrodisiac – a substance claimed to enhance sexual desire or performance

Deliriant – a hallucinogenic compound with dissociative effects

Depressant – a substance that reduces stimulation

Dissociative – producing sensations of detachment from the body

DMT – dimethyltryptamine, a hallucinatory substance

Empathogen – a substance that increases one's social/emotional awareness

Entheogen – a psychoactive substance usually taken in a spiritual or religious context

Ethnobotany – the study of the relationship between people and plants

Ethnomycology – the study of how people use fungi and its significance in cultures

Euphoriant – a substance that stimulates euphoria

Fumagatory – a plant used for its smoke-producing qualities

Hallucinogen – a psychoactive substance used to alter the sense of perception, mood or consciousness

Masticatory – a plant that is mainly chewed

MDMA – Methylenedioxymethamphetamine, a recreational drug also known as ecstasy

Mescaline – a psychedelic substance, found in certain cacti

Narcotics – drugs that suppress the functions of the brain leading to a state of torpor or unconsciousness

Psilocybin – a psychedelic substance commonly found in *Psilocybe* species of mushrooms

Psychedelia – the art and culture associated with psychedelic experiences

Psychedelic – a class of drugs that alter consciousness, often inducing hallucinations, including visual, aural or olfactory stimulation

Psychoactive – mind-altering

Psychonaut – a slang term for someone who uses entheogenic substances for exploring the mind

Psychotropic – a substance that affects the brain, altering emotions, awareness and/or behaviour

Stimulant – a substance that increases brain activity

Opposite An illustration of *Camellia sinensis*.

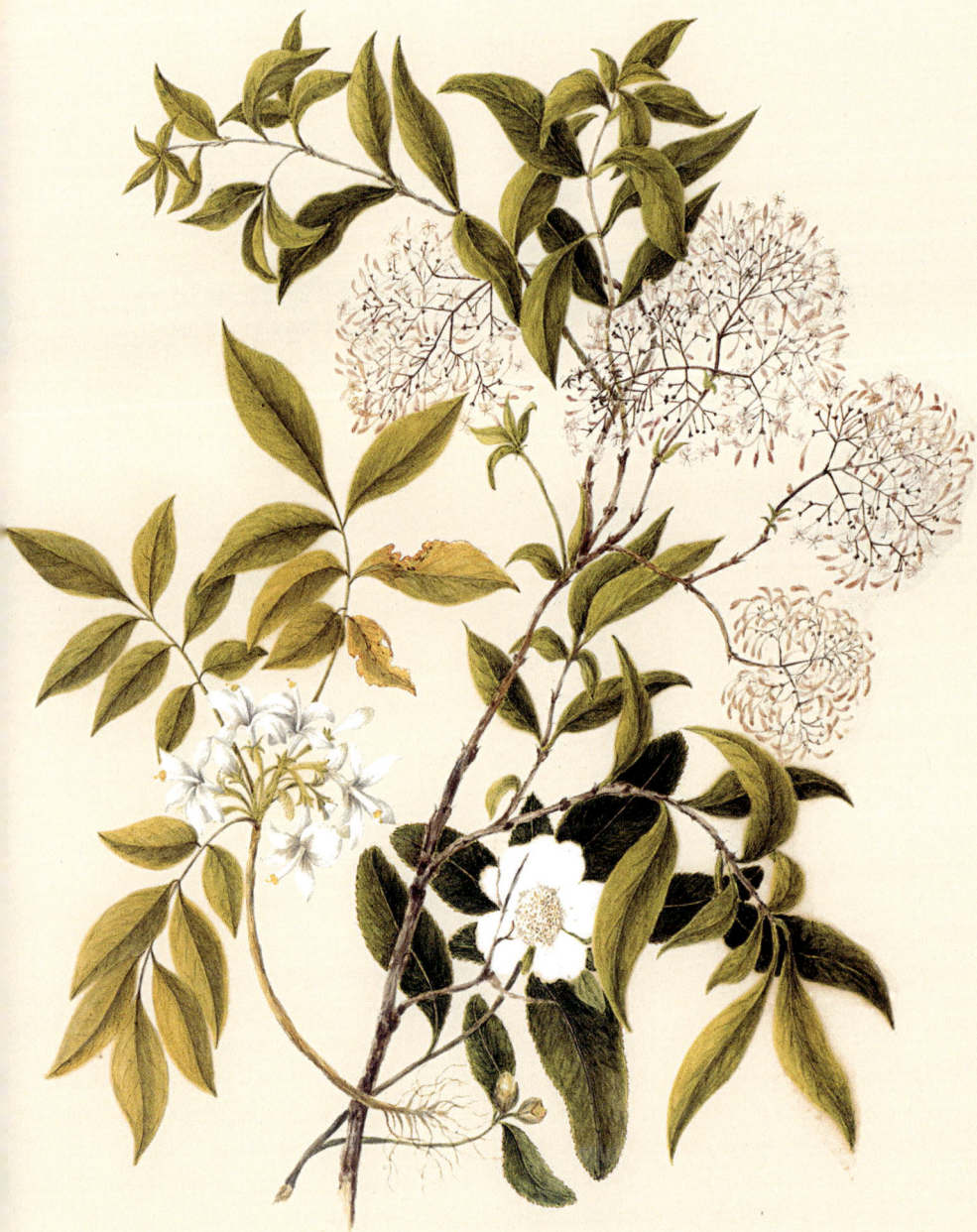

Further Reading

A s with all the volumes in this series, it is impossible in a book this size to cover every possible aspect of the folklore, superstition or, in particular, the popular culture around its subject, psychoactive plants.

Any number of superb books, articles, journals, websites and other, less tangible, sources, often about a specific substance, or even a specific aspect of a specific substance, have been part of the process of distilling such an enormous subject into so very few pages. A snippet here, a mention there; rabbit holes have been jumped down, wild geese chased and better brains than my own consulted – not least those of Dr Melanie-Jayne Howes, Senior Research Leader in Biological Chemistry; Initiative Leader in Biointeractions and Bioactive Molecules at the Royal Botanic Gardens, Kew. I must also thank Mary Lawrence, a student of Cha Dao, for her insights into the world of living tea, much more complex than I had imagined.

As always, I consulted far too many works to cite in full, but listed below are a few I found particularly and consistently helpful, offered as possible starting points for further research into this labyrinthine and often confusing world.

Dr Howes's own work, written with Elizabeth A. Dauncey, *Plants that Cure: Plants as a Source of Medicines, from Pharmaceuticals to Herbal Remedies* (Royal Botanic Gardens, Kew, 2020), mainly covers the medicinal properties of plants, but often strays into the psychoactive world. *Plants that Heal, Thrill and Kill*, by Wee Yeow Chin (SNP, 2005), also

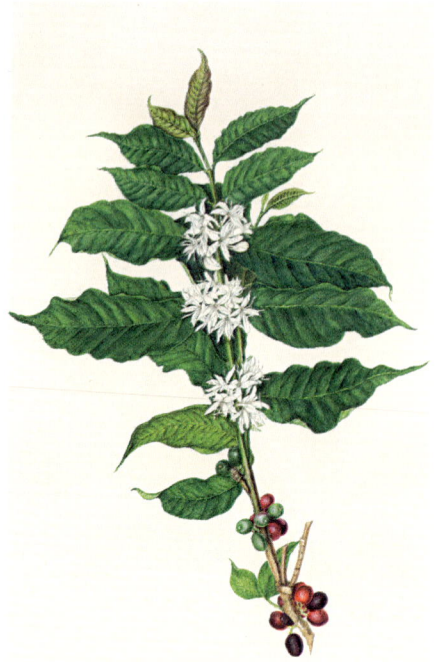

Above An illustration of *Coffea arabica*.

discusses a range of intoxicating plants alongside those that either kill you or make you better.

Mike Jay's *Psychonauts: Drugs and the Making of the Modern Mind* (Yale University Press, 2022) was one of several works that provided an excellent overview of the subject, but sometimes it was necessary to drill down into a specific substance. I turned to Alistair Hay, Monika Gottshalk and Adolfo Holguin's *Huanduj: The Genus Brugmansia* (Royal Botanic Gardens, Kew, 2012) and Daniel Pinchbeck and

Sophia Rokhlin's *When Plants Dream: Ayahuasca, Amazonian Shamanism and the Global Psychedelic Renaissance* (Watkins Publishing, 2021).

Wicked Plants: The A–Z of Plants that Kill, Maim, Intoxicate and Otherwise Offend by Amy Stewart (Timber Press, 2010) includes some curious stories about intoxicating plants that overlap with poisons, while Cody Johnson's *Magic Medicine: A Trip through the Intoxicating History and Modern-Day Use of Psychedelic Plants and Substances* (Fair Winds Press, 2018) makes the science work, writing with historical authority and genuine wit. It's worth checking out his website, too: psychedelicfrontier.com

As far as practical works are concerned, I heartily thank the mysterious Raisa Sinclair for *A Field Guide to Deliriants* (2019) which takes the reader through a minute-by-minute account as the author ingests some of the wackier hallucinogens so that we don't have to.

There are certain folkloric works without which I never set out on a new cultural journey, including Vickery's *Folk Flora: an A–Z of the Folklore and Uses of British and Irish Plants* (Weidenfeld & Nicolson, 2019), and I am always keen to see what folklore author, podcaster and blogger Icy Sedgwick has

to say about a subject: see icysedgwick.com

Sarah Penicka's scholarly article, 'Caveat Anoynter!: A Study of Flying Ointments and their Plants' (*The Dark Side: Proceedings of the Seventh Australian and International Religion, Literature and the Arts Conference*, 2002, RLA Press, 2004) gave me much pause for thought, as did the excellent exhibition *Why Do We Take Drugs?* at the Sainsbury Centre, University of East Anglia, Norwich.

Particularly useful in terms of the pop culture surrounding the subject were *The Hip: Hipsters, Jazz and the Beat Generation*, by Roy Carr, Brian Case and Fred Dellar (Faber & Faber, 1987) and Max Décharné's *Straight From The Fridge, Dad: A Dictionary of Hipster Slang* (No Exit Press, 2000). Łukasz Kamieński's *Shooting Up: A History of Drugs in Warfare* (Hurst, 2016) was invaluable, and not just for exploring war on drugs.

The single most useful work of all for this particular book, however, was, by far, the seminal *Plants of the Gods: Their Sacred, Healing, and Hallucinogenic Powers*, by Richard Evans Schultes, Albert Hofmann and Cristian Rätsch, particularly useful in its revised edition of 1992.

Index

Credits

The publishers would like to thank the following sources for their kind permission to reproduce the pictures in this book.

All other images are from the Library and Archives collection of the Royal Botanic Gardens, Kew.

ADOBE STOCK: 147

AKG-IMAGES: Interfoto 90

ALAMY STOCK PHOTO: Nataliia Babkina 140; Neil Baylis 65; Contraband Collection 111; Malcolm Fairman 187; FlixPix 156; Granger - Historical Picture Archive 116; Chris Howes / Wild Places Photography 37; Natalia Lukiianova 13; John Mitchell 182; Pictorial Press Ltd 76; The Picture Art Collection 11; Retro AdArchives 151, 160; SBS Eclectic Images 152; Philip Scalia 134; SilverScreen 155; Vintage_Space 33

BRIDGEMAN IMAGES: Archives Charmet 86; Florilegius (chapter openers); Imagebroker (chapter openers); Pictures from History 38; The Stapleton Collection (chapter openers)

CREATIVE COMMONS: 121

ILLUSTRATIONS COMMISSIONED BY MALCOLM ENGLISH: 143, 185

GETTY IMAGES: Bettmann 49, 112, 125; DeAgostini 12, 170; GAB Archive / Redferns 148; Hulton Archive 89; ivan-96 / DigitalVision Vectors 14; John Kobal Foundation 69; Mykhailo Melnychenko / Babel / Global Images Ukraine 105; The San Francisco Chronicle 129; Sean Sexton / Hulton Archive 66

MARY EVANS PICTURE LIBRARY: 61, 79, 80; Everett Collection 122; Photo Researchers 21; Retrograph Collection 41; Weimar Archive 104

SHUTTERSTOCK: Granger 107; lamnee 29; Talita Santana Campos 136-137

WELLCOME COLLECTION: 117

WIKIMEDIA CREATIVE COMMONS: 53, 139, 165; New York Public Library 64

Published in 2026 by Welbeck
An Imprint of HEADLINE PUBLISHING GROUP LIMITED

1

Cataloguing in Publication Data is available from the British Library

ISBN 9781035422227

Printed and bound in Dubai by Oriental Press

MIX
Paper | Supporting
responsible forestry
FSC
www.fsc.org
FSC® C104740

Headline's policy is to use papers that are natural, renewable and recyclable products and made from wood grown in well-managed forests and other controlled sources. The logging and manufacturing processes are expected to conform to the environmental regulations of the country of origin.

HEADLINE PUBLISHING GROUP LIMITED
An Hachette UK Company
Carmelite House
50 Victoria Embankment
London EC4Y 0DZ

The authorized representative in the EEA is Hachette Ireland,
8 Castlecourt Centre, Dublin 15, D15 XTP3, Ireland
(email: info@hbgi.ie)

www.headline.co.uk
www.hachette.co.uk